CW00918911

The Wellness

Om Swami is a mystic who lives in the Himalayan foothills. An advanced yogin, Swami has done thousands of hours of intense meditation in complete seclusion in Himalayan caves and woods.

Prior to renunciation, he founded and ran a multi million-dollar software company with offices in San Francisco, New York, Toronto, London, Sydney and India. Om Swami has a bachelor's degree in business and an MBA from Sydney, Australia. He completely renounced his business interests a few years ago to pursue a full-time spiritual life.

He is also the author of the best-selling *If Truth be Told: A Monk's Memoir*. You can connect with him on his blog, omswami.com, which is read by millions all over the world.

The Wellness Sense

A Practical Guide to Your Physical and Emotional Health Based on Ayurvedic and Yogic Wisdom

OM SWAMI

First published in India in 2015 by Harper Element
An imprint of HarperCollins *Publishers*

Worldwide publishing rights: Black Lotus Press

Copyright © Om Swami 2015

P-ISBN: 978-0-9940027-3-0
E-ISBN: 978-0-9940027-0-9

Om Swami asserts the moral right to be identified as the
author of this work.
www.omswami.com

The views and opinions expressed in this book are the
author's own and the facts are as reported by him, and
the publishers are not in any way liable for the same.

This work is not a substitute for treatment or advice by a
qualified health care professional.

All rights reserved. No part of this publication may be
reproduced, stored in a retrieval system, or transmitted,
in any form or by any means, electronic, mechanical,
photocopying, recording or otherwise, without the prior
permission of the publishers.

This work is dedicated
to the welfare of all sentient beings

Om pūrṇamadaḥ pūrṇamidaṁ pūrṇātpurṇamudacyate,
Pūrṇasya pūrṇamādāya pūrṇamevāvaśiṣyate.

That is complete. This is complete. From complete
has emerged complete. After taking complete
away from complete, what remains is also
complete.
(Peace chant, *Ishavasya Upanishad*.)

We, who have emerged from nature, from God,
are complete in every sense of the word.

Acknowledgements

When I wrote this book, it was extremely important for me to have my views validated by qualified medical professionals. I wanted to provide you authentic information that you could rely on, and not just a figment of my imagination. Because what you have in your hands is not merely an introduction to Ayurveda, but a detailed exposition of the collective wisdom contained in Ayurvedic and yogic scriptures. I wanted to eliminate even the slightest possibility of overrating my own experiences or misinterpreting medical texts in any way. To this effect, I am deeply indebted to the following brilliant and busy doctors, who not only took time out of their hectic schedules to read my manuscript but also provided comprehensive and insightful feedback:

Vivek Tripathi, MBBS
Renu Madan, BHMS
Jayavani Pandey, BAMS
Ravi Verma, MD
Priyanka Sara, MD

R.C. Pandey, MD
Chetana Verma, MD
L. Mahadevan, MD
I would like to thank the commissioning editor at HarperCollins, Ajitha G.S., who not only agreed to publish this book so that it reaches a wider audience, but also personally reviewed the manuscript offering wonderful and candid feedback along the way.

I would specially like to thank Sameer Mahale, national sales manager, at HarperCollins who saw the promise in this book and worked hard to ensure that it is released well within 2015.

Also, I can't thank enough my first editor, Ismita Tandon, for doing a magnificent job with the early draft of my work.

I'm equally grateful to some very kind people, notably, John Coen, Camila Vicenci, Jocelyn Meli and Shaun Jenkins, who went the extra mile and gave me detailed feedback.

My gratitude to Garima Om and Anju Modgil for going over the manuscript with impeccable attention to detail, reviewing each and every word.

I would also like to thank Carl A. Harte for his thoughtful review, and Rea Mukherjee for the final scan.

My gratitude to Saurabh Garge at HarperCollins for the beautiful cover design.

And, above all, my deepest gratitude to Mother Nature for using me as an instrument and allowing the ancient wisdom to flow through.

Contents

About This Book

In these pages, I have combined my reflections on major Ayurvedic texts with my years of experience in yoga and tantra, to give you the essence of health and well-being. To make the most out of this book, read it patiently as if chewing gum, to enjoy and absorb the knowledge contained herein.

Although I received my formal education in information technology and business, for years I have practised healing and experimented across the disciplines of astrology, mantra, tantra, meditation and alchemy. While Ayurvedic texts mostly focus on physical health, and yogic scriptures on mental well-being, tantric scriptures pay attention to the metaphysical aspects of our existence.

When we synthesize the wisdom across the three disciplines of Ayurveda, yoga and tantra, we gain a unique and holistic understanding of health. Because all three insist that we are an integral part of nature, anything that happens in the play of nature affects us. Therefore, the more you are in harmony with nature, the more peaceful and healthy you will be. The objective of this book is to help you see how your body – your health and well-being – is intricately linked to Mother Nature, and how living in harmony with nature brings changes in your own nature.

I have always been passionate about health and natural remedies. So much so, I once owned an Ayurvedic health care company with a research team comprising some of the most brilliant Ayurvedic doctors in India. During the clinical trials of our products, I had the opportunity to meet and interview many patients. Except for Vishy's example (in Chapter 6), all case studies in this book are real. I have only changed the names and, at times, places to protect the privacy of the individuals concerned. I have mostly used the masculine pronoun in general references for convenience purposes only; the teachings of Ayurveda and yoga are universally applicable.

I hope this book motivates you to lead a more natural, healthier and more peaceful life.

Introduction

Even though I grew up reading Ayurvedic, yogic and tantric scriptures expounding on health, yoga and alchemy, my own health was never good. For the greater part of my life, as a patient of asthma, I was allergic to pollen. I don't remember a change of season when I didn't fall sick. I was living proof of modern medicine's belief that allergies could only be treated temporarily. I had given up my asthma medication with the help of a controlled diet. Yet, every year, at the dawn of spring, my asthma would get worse and I would start gobbling up cough syrups and cold and flu tablets. With a red nose, heavy head and a wheezing chest, I would increase the dosage of my inhalers and lose most of my appetite.

My body needed rest, but time was perhaps the one thing I could not afford. My projects, teams and clients needed me every day, in five different time zones, and the immense stress at work left me gasping for breath. Exercising at the gym, playing badminton, eating organic food and taking supplements only helped a little. The fact remained that whenever seasons changed, I fell sick. I would notice those who remained mostly healthy, regardless of the pressure at work or the challenges at home they endured. Many of these healthy people even ate unhealthily, yet they remained mostly fit. I seriously wondered: 'What is the secret to their health?' There is no secret, really. In accordance with Ayurveda, I came to the conclusion that each one of us is truly different, and some of us are more prone to certain diseases than others. I accepted the fact that asthma was my way of life.

A few years later, however, I renounced the material world and went to the Himalayas to begin my life as a monk. I stayed in the woods and caves for nearly thirteen months, and while there, I didn't even so much as contract a common cold, let alone any major ailments or asthma. Surviving on one frugal meal a day – and sometimes just on snow – when I emerged from my hut many months later after intense meditation, I felt fitter and stronger than ever before. I meditated in open fields during spring and in caves during winters, yet there was no sign of any allergy.

I had never felt this before: being completely free of any physical ailments for months at a stretch. This experience challenged my earlier conclusion. I figured that it's never too late to take control of your well-being and, no matter what your genetic disposition, you can attain near-perfect health. Having said that, I observed that we, as a human race, fall ill more frequently and for longer durations than any other species. The animals we have tamed also fall sick more often than their wild counterparts.

I reflected on my perfect health in the Himalayas and figured that there were many factors contributing to my well-being there. I realized that living in harmony with nature and adopting some of the yogic principles were the primary reasons why I did not fall sick at all. I examined the truths of Ayurvedic and yogic scriptures in a new light now. Just Ayurvedic concoctions, some yogasanas or tantric practices alone, were not sufficient to cure my illness. The key was to combine all of them. But, most notably, what had worked was leading a simple life in the most natural way. While in the woods, I was in constant touch with Mother Nature, and her incredible healing powers brought about profound changes in my body and mind.

I do understand that many of us can't afford to leave the hustle and bustle of the town even for a day, let alone go away and live in the woods for months. It is for this reason that I have written this book, because this is what is remarkable about Ayurveda and yoga: you do not have to live in the woods or in the Himalayas to be in touch with nature. An entire cosmos exists within you. You do not have to be flexible like a rubber doll either, because I won't be asking you to assume any complicated postures. You just need the willingness to understand health in its entirety, and the discipline to take control of your physical and emotional well-being.

Our body is the finest, in fact the only, medium of experiencing all pleasures and sorrows. In Ayurveda, as in yoga and tantra, the health of an individual is not just the state of his physical body but an aggregate of the body, senses, mind and soul. Your immune system is directly impacted by your state of mind. The more positive and happy you are, the stronger your immunity.

According to Ayurveda, health and disease have the same source. When various entities (covered later in this book) are in harmony, it translates into health. And when they are in disequilibrium, they cause disorders. Your body is merely the seat of your consciousness. If your consciousness is afflicted, it will surely – without exception – result in physical disorders too. Mental afflictions create diseases in the physical body and physical diseases, in turn, disturb the state of mind.

More often than not, an unhealthy mental state is the cause of illness – particularly with adults. You can treat the disease in the physical body, but that's merely treating the symptom. Such a disease will recur. For example, you can take anti-allergy medication to avoid hay fever, but it will come back every year. To remain disease-free, it is important to have a healthy mind and a healthy body; they complement each other. And attaining a healthy body and healthy mind is the core philosophy of Ayurveda.

The modern system of medicine is mostly symptom-driven. If I have a headache, it'll tell me to take a painkiller. Ayurveda does not believe in treating symptoms. It advocates understanding the patient and treating the cause of the symptom and not the symptom itself. In order to do this, the ancient scriptures take a far more holistic approach to health by taking into account our lifestyle combined with our natural tendencies (which vary from one person to another). In other words, it understands that one man's medicine could be another man's poison. Yogurt, for example, may aid digestion in some people but cause indigestion in others.

Further, just focussing on your physical health by way of better diet and exercise is only a fraction of the solution. The important part is taking care of your mental and emotional health. How you respond to what life throws at you affects your health in the most significant manner. You cannot choose your parents, your siblings, your country of birth and so forth. You cannot change your boss, your spouse, your children or your friends. The economy, the country and the state of society is largely beyond your control. You may have a few, if any, practical choices in these. You can, however, choose how you feel about those elements of your life and how you respond to them. The way you look at anything and the manner in which you accept or react are the two most important – if not the only – factors that determine your overall well-being. If you can either change your perspective or your response towards what you find disturbing, ninety per cent of the job is done. The remaining ten per cent is simply about body fitness. Yogic wisdom helps you gain mental equilibrium and Ayurveda, physical well-being.

Yogic texts believe that as bliss is the natural state of your mind, health is the natural state of your body. When your mind is in its natural state, you feel peaceful naturally. Similarly, when your body is in its natural state – when the various constituents of your body, like humours (dosha), tissues (dhatu), digestive fire (agni), and energy flow (vayu) are in equilibrium – you are disease-free; you are healthy. Any thought that disturbs your mental balance is a negative thought even if it is about God. Conversely, any thought that gives you peace is a positive thought. The more you fill your mind with positive thoughts, the better your state of mind will be. And that naturally results in better physical health.

The Sanskrit word for health is svasthya; it means self-dependence or a sound state of the body and mind. If examined further, it means your natural state: sva means natural, and sthya means state or place. Ayurveda aims to restore your natural state, your balance, so you may be free of mental and physical afflictions.

I've had patients successfully cure ulcers, cancers, migraines, obesity, hypertension, allergies, depression and many other ailments, by following the principles I share with you in this book. I am not suggesting that Ayurveda is a panacea. No system of medicine is. But when you combine the principles of Ayurveda with yogic thought, you make a giant leap in your understanding of the human body and its well-being. In this book, I introduce to you a holistic system of health and wellness.

My goal is not to give you herbal remedies, because once again I don't wish to treat symptoms. Besides, I'm not a medical professional but a meditation specialist and a tantric practitioner. There are plenty of Ayurvedic doctors out there whom you can consult for medicine. Having said that, the chances are that, once you adopt the principles and practices I am sharing here, you will not need to see a doctor again. For a healthy and long life, ancient yogic thought offers to you one of the most insightful, complete and scientific perspectives.

I promise, by the time you finish reading this book, you will look upon your body and your health in a new way. You will learn how to take better care of yourself; you will know how to lead a healthier life in our present world – a world where we have all the comforts yet we are restless. We have organic breakfast on the table but no time to eat it; we have the most comfortable mattresses but little sleep. The key to wholesome living and well-being is entirely in your hands. You alone can take control of your physical and emotional health. Let me show you how.

2

Mother Nature and Your Body

I had known Jay, a man in his early forties, for many years. He was a migrant from India and was living in Canada. Jay had been a vegetarian for more than a decade. He went to the gym three times a week, lived a life of moderation and played squash regularly. He occasionally meditated too. His previous partner had left him without any warning, but he was now happily married. Jay had no major stresses in life and no debts, and while he was not entirely satisfied with his career, he was an IT professional and made good money.

Except for a sensitive stomach, and therefore occasional episodes of indigestion, he had no health problems. Before he contacted me, Jay had suffered from hay fever on account of a seasonal allergy. It had triggered bouts of coughing and a blocked nose. A few days later the nose was no longer runny or blocked, but the cough continued. Thinking it was merely the seasonal allergy, he avoided going to the doctor and took off-the-shelf cough syrups and tablets instead. Two weeks went by, and the cough persisted. Finally, he went to his family doctor, who prescribed some medication.

There was no improvement though, and he started feeling feverish too. His wife noticed slight swelling around his neck with soft lumps. There was absolutely no pain. He thought it was just the extended hay fever weighing him down. The cough didn't improve, the fever didn't go down and the swelling stayed. Again, he consulted his doctor, who prescribed some tests including blood tests. A few days later, he was recommended to a specialist.

The pathologist took a sample from one of the lumps and sent it to a lab. Three days later he was back in the specialist's clinic. Both he and the specialist had something to show the other. Jay showed him more lumps in his armpits and groin. They were growing quickly. And the specialist showed him his biopsy report. He had Hodgkin's lymphoma, a cancer of the lymph nodes. Further tests showed that the lumps were also growing in his chest. High-dose chemotherapy was recommended immediately, followed by radiation therapy. It was a Friday and the first session of chemotherapy was scheduled for Tuesday. This was when Jay called me and apprised me of the situation for the first time. He wanted to know if there was an alternative.

I needed at least six weeks to try anything, and three weeks was the absolute bare minimum, because any yogic, tantric or Ayurvedic remedy requires that long to work. I told him that diseases in the physical body were merely an expression of our consciousness and, if his doctor was willing to move the chemotherapy by at least three weeks, we could try an alternative treatment. He said he would speak to the doctor and find out if it was possible. In the meantime, I asked him to get in touch with an Ayurvedic physician I really trusted. The physician was in India and Jay was in Canada. Ayurveda would take care of his physical body, and I recommended him a meditation, a yogic practice and a tantric practice to work on the subtler aspects of his disease.

The only other ingredient I required for his healing was faith, which was not lacking, because Jay had known me for years. I needed faith because it connects at the deepest level of your existence. It transcends the talkative mind and the calculative mind and goes straight through to your soul. We asked the Ayurvedic physician to immediately courier the drugs, anyway. On Monday, Jay called me and said he had bought additional time, and his high-dose chemotherapy was now scheduled to commence three weeks later.

He started with the two practices and meditation right away, and by Thursday he was taking his Ayurvedic medicine. Three weeks later he saw his specialist. There was no cough, no fever and no swelling. There were no lumps at all. The specialist was at his wit's end. Tests were conducted again, and the severity of the disease had decreased by more than ninety-five per cent. The doctor gave Jay the option of going ahead with chemotherapy. It would be light chemo, with one session every six weeks and no radiation therapy was required, he was told.

I told Jay I couldn't possibly take a call on whether he should forego chemo completely, because I wasn't a medical professional or a cancer specialist. Our Ayurvedic physician stated that light chemo was the right thing to do and that it would do no harm. I asked Jay to continue with the meditation and the other two practices. Not only did Jay keep all his hair during the chemotherapy, he actually gained healthy weight; he felt and looked fitter than ever before. Nearly a decade has elapsed since, and all is well with Jay.

The only real difference between the specialist's and my thinking was in our perspectives. He had been trained to see physical diseases as the originator of all infections and ailments. I, on the other hand, belonged to the old school. I don't see diseases in the physical body as the cause; I see them as a manifestation of an anomaly in the consciousness. Most physical ailments have a deep-rooted cause that is not in the physical body. In Jay's case, it was his sense of betrayal and anger towards his former partner. Further in this book, in the chapter 'Mental Afflictions', I touch upon how emotions like anger harm our health.

So, what is the human body made of? What comes to your mind when you think of your body? Is it just a holder of flesh, bones and blood? The physical body you see on the outside is merely one aspect of you. Your body is a conglomerate of a myriad of elements that work together to make it what it is. Not all of those elements are physical, but they are all perceptible. We can touch and feel various body parts. We can examine and hold all the physical elements. But beyond the physical, there are other forces at play. For example, we can't touch or hold our thoughts, but they can make us feel a certain way; they can have a positive or a negative impact on our physical health. We can't even touch our own breath – which is the very basis of our existence. The subtler elements require greater sensitivity of the consciousness.

Your physical health is almost entirely dependent on how your body accepts and processes food, which in turn is affected by your mental and emotional state. The body is not just a mechanical machine, for if it were, all stomachs would process food exactly the same way. The truth is that everyone's body is unique. Even if two people eat identical meals, their bodies respond to them differently. What is that factor, that element, that thing in their bodies that determines how they are going to process food?

Einstein used to say, 'It's not that I'm smarter, it's just that I stay with problems longer.' Yogis in ancient India gained remarkable insights into the nature of human existence based on the same principle – they meditated on it for long periods. Gradually, their insights were refined and evolved into a concrete system, complete with an underlying theory and a set of practices, most of which are scientifically verifiable even today.

They divided the primary aspects of our wellness into the physical and mental. Ayurveda covered the physical aspects and yogic scriptures expounded the mental aspects. The four key physical ones are: pancha-bhoota (the five elements), sapta-dhatu (the seven tissues), tri-dosha (the three humours), and chatush-agni (the four fires). The four key mental aspects are: pancha-kosha (the five sheaths), tri-guna (the three mental states), tri-kaya (the three bodies), and dasa-vayu (the ten energies). Information on the five sheaths, three bodies and ten vital energies can be found in the appendix of this book. The remaining aspects are covered in appropriate sections.

Whether you want to lose or gain weight, whether you want to look younger or be more virile, remain free of diseases and afflictions or just be physically stronger, a complete understanding of your body is the starting point. Without further ado, let me get to the heart of the matter, beginning with the five elements.

THE FIVE GREAT ELEMENTS

Harmony means balance; it means equilibrium. It is impossible to fall sick if you are in equilibrium. Everything in nature, including our body, is made up of five elements. They are called pancha maha-bhoota in Sanskrit. It means the five great elements. They are called earth, water, fire, air and ether. The more you are in touch with your elements, the more you are in harmony with Mother Nature.

The closer you are to nature, the healthier you remain and the quicker you recover from any disorders. In the woods, still untouched by humans or their cattle, I never saw a sick or dying plant. Once I started to go into areas inhabited by humans, I saw many plants suffering from one disease or the other. It is our artificial lifestyle that drives us away from nature and its healing powers, and creates illnesses. The five great elements make us an intrinsic part of nature.

Everything outside your body is a part of the macrocosm. You are an exact replica of that macrocosm. Just like there's a universe outside, there's a universe inside. Only the quantity varies; the quality doesn't. Vedic texts refer to the human body as the microcosm. Macrocosm is called brahmanda. It means an egg of the primordial force. And the microcosm is called pindanda. It means an egg of a part of the whole. Each entity in nature is complete in its own right. A drop of water and an ocean have exactly the same properties. Qualitatively speaking, they are identical. An ocean may have infinite number of drops, but each drop is complete in its own right. An ocean too is one giant drop of water. Similarly, when we get in touch with nature, our tiny existence taps into the enormous and infinite forces of nature, and we automatically gain health and bliss.

There is, therefore, a close and intricately correlating relationship between our well-being and our universe. Around seventy per cent of the earth's surface is water-covered; your body is approximately seventy per cent water. There are infinite stars in the sky; there are countless pores on your body. There is the milky way; you have the lymphatic system. There are rivers, small and large, merging into the oceans that further represent one giant waterbody; there are arteries and veins in your body ending in your heart. Air is the fundamental life ingredient on this planet; it is the basic need of your body. There is space around you; there is space in each of the nine orifices – or ten orifices in the case of females – in your body. Whatever you can find in the macrocosm, you can find inside your body.

Absolutely everything is made up of the five great elements. Yogic texts offer simple characteristics of these elements. Earth is hard and stable. Water is fluid and flexible. Fire is vital warmth and a transformative force. Air represents motion and flow. Ether or space is the entire body, most notably the pores and orifices. These five elements are linked to the five sense objects and five forms of consciousness and the five organs. See the table below:

The Five Elements and Our Body

Element	Consciousness	Organ	Perception
Earth	Olfactive	Nostrils	Smell
Water	Gustative	Tongue	Taste
Fire	Visual	Eyes	Form
Air	Tactual	Skin	Touch
Ether	Auditive	Ears	Sound

The five elements don't just correspond to the five sensory objects. They are not just about the physical composition of your body; they are more than that. For example, purification of each element positively affects its corresponding consciousness, organ and perception.

Beyond just the sensory organs and resultant perception, tantric texts link the five elements to various aspects of our health and body. Hair, skin, nails, flesh and bones are made from the earth element. People born with a dominant earth element tend to be stout or have a heavy skeletal structure. They are more stable-minded than the other four types. An impure earth element can cause diseases of the skin, flesh or bones. It can lead to great restlessness.

Urine, stools, marrow, blood and semen are governed by the water element. An impure water element often leads to diseases of the reproductive organs. When both water and fire are impure, it causes hypertension (high blood pressure), and when both water and air are impure, it causes hypotension (low blood pressure), for example.

Laziness, fatigue, thirst, hunger and sleep are the characteristics of the fire element. Purification of the fire element has a direct and immediate bearing on one's hunger and laziness. When I was in the woods for months at a stretch, I required only two hours of sleep and one meal each day. For the rest of the time, I meditated with awareness and alertness. There were times when I felt tired due to extreme physical and mental exertion, but never did I feel fatigued, hungry or sleepy. This was particularly on account of purification of the fire element, as part of my meditational and tantric routine.

Expansion, contraction, release, movement and holding are governed by the air element. Therefore, strength and agility of the limbic system is greatly influenced by the dominance and purity of the air element. Further, impurity of the air element is responsible for most neurological disorders in our bodies. Purification of this element strengthens the central nervous system, and lends strength and suppleness to the limbs.

Greed, fear, attachment, anger and desire are the characteristics of the ether element. It is mostly on account of these five that we bring suffering upon ourselves. When any of these is present, there is no contentment; there is no peace. Impurity or dominance of the ether element creates most emotional disorders.

The science of Ayurveda predominantly focuses on the earth, water and the fire elements. Yogic practices enhance the first three, and in addition, purify the air and the ether elements. Tantra makes extensive use of both Ayurvedic and yogic practices, whether that is doing special worship, making fire offerings, performing rituals, anointing the body, consuming mixtures or even smoking weed. Alchemy is an integral part of tantra. It was first practised by tantriks, long before the concept of medicine was known to the average person.

Purification of the elements is a remarkable tantric practice called bhoota shuddhi. It is a powerful visualization to purify your elemental body for better physical and mental health. By purifying each element, the practitioner can eliminate the diseases linked to that element. This practice is passed in disciplic succession from a tantrik guru to the initiated disciple. I can tell you from my personal experience that purification of the elements takes your wellness to a whole new level. For now, let me elaborate on the seven tissues – the heart of Ayurveda.

THE SEVEN TISSUES

Your physical body is made up of seven key constituents. These constituents are different forms of body tissues, called sapta-dhatu: the seven tissues or secretions. Before I elaborate on them, it is important to understand the word dhatu. One standard meaning of dhatu is constituent. In the context of Ayurveda, it is understood as body tissue. The word dhatu in Sanskrit also means the primary element. The food you eat is made up of the five great elements. Once food is processed by your body, it is broken down to form the seven dhatus. These are the bodily elements, primary constituents that are the building blocks of the physical body. From the Sanskrit root dha, dhatu also means to possess, to accept, to bestow. How your body accepts the food you consume, directly determines the quality of your health. Additionally, dhatu means secretion.

An embryo is formed because the parents secrete an egg and a sperm. The fetus survives because the mother secretes through the umbilical cord. Once out in the world, the infant survives because his mother's breasts are secreting milk. As he grows, he can chew food because certain glands are secreting saliva. The food is digested because the intestinal glands are secreting. The human body is made up of secretions. As per Ayurveda, anything we consume, our body breaks down into seven dhatus or secretions. These are the body's primary constituents. Ayurveda has put them in the following order, because it was believed that each subsequent secretion is harder for the body to manufacture and maintain.

Rasa

The English word for rasa is chyle. As with any language, however, there are certain words in Sanskrit that have no equivalent in English. Rasa is one such word. The taste in food is rasa; the fluid in anything is rasa; the melody in music is rasa; visual beauty is rasa; the feeling of success is rasa and the emotion in an orgasm is rasa. It also means juice or sap. Further, rasa refers to a body tissue, and most notably, blood plasma.

Rasa is the first stage of any food consumed by the body. Before it converts into nutrients usable by the body, it must first become liquid in the intestine.

Blood

Blood, the second dhatu, is called rakta in Sanskrit. Rakta refers to the red blood cells, the haemoglobin and the blood platelets. Although the science of Ayurveda did not categorize blood into cells, platelets and haemoglobin, it did indeed understand that blood had certain constituents that allowed it to flow, to nourish and to clot. The word rakta, if split as ra + akta, means that which is characteristic of heat. Akta also means oil. Rakta is the substance that is living as long as it has the constituents that retain its innate heat and fluidity. Ra also means love. The desire and act of lovemaking causes a rush of blood in the blood vessels; it raises the body temperature (heat is blood's innate property). Like all the other dhatus, blood is absolutely essential to human existence.

Muscle

Mamsa is the third dhatu. It means muscle or flesh. It is interesting to note that Ayurveda specifically differentiated between muscle and fat (the next dhatu). Even five thousand years ago, its practitioners well understood the difference between the two. The basic building block of muscle is protein.

Fat

Meda is the fourth dhatu. It means fat – in particular, the adipose tissue in your body. The joints in the body are lubricated by a synovial fluid. It is a viscid lubricating fluid in the joints, tendon sheaths and capsular ligaments surrounding the joints. But in Ayurveda, meda not only refers to the adipose tissue but also to the synovial fluid. Meda allows your body to retain its warmth. Its primary seat is the torso.

Bones

The fifth dhatu is referred to as asthi, meaning bones. This is the supporting structure of your body. Ayurvedic texts consider teeth as bones too.

Marrow

Majja is the sixth dhatu. It means marrow. It is the network of tissues that fills the cavities of a bone. The word medha (not to be confused with meda which means fat, the fourth dhatu) is a synonym of majja. Interestingly, the word for mental vigour is medhaa. Do you see the connection? Even though the brain is a muscle, it is enclosed in bone – the skull – just like bone marrow. Therefore, according to Ayurveda, anything that nourishes your bone marrow will also nourish your brain.

Shukra

Like the word rasa, shukra connotes more than its literal meaning. Hence, I've chosen to use the Sanskrit term. Generally, shukra means semen. In Ayurveda, it is used to mean the reproductive fluids of both men and women. The female sexual fluids are also called artava (lit: menstrual blood) or shonita (lit: blood). Ayurveda didn't have the sophisticated testing methods available today to ascertain that it was not the blood, but hormones like oestrogen and progesterone, that are the true sexual fluids. Nevertheless, it understood that a woman's sexual fluids were quite different from a man's.

Further – and somewhat surprisingly – Vedic texts state that a sperm joins with an egg to form a fetus – a statement perfectly in line with the modern view. Shukra has been put last on the list of the dhatus. Yogic texts do not consider shukra to be a mere reproductive fluid. They call it the creative fluid; it is virility in men and fertility in women.

One's mental (intelligence), physical (body growth) and biological (procreation) creativity depends on the well-being of the first six dhatus. Ayurvedic texts consider the male sexual fluid to have thermolytic properties (soma-guna), whereas the female sexual fluid is considered to have thermogenic characteristics (agni-guna). Soma means soothing, cool, and agni means fire, thermal. Therefore, after the act of sexual intercourse, a man loses body heat and is ready to rest or fall asleep, but a woman generally becomes more active, or hungry. She feels relaxed too, but her reproductive fluid is of a different nature – it rouses her sensory perception and tends to make her more aware and alert.

Shukra also means light, bright and pure. Light is a synonym of wisdom in Sanskrit. It directly means that a life of purity, lived with discerning wisdom, ensures the complete well-being of a person.

I took the time to cover the core concepts of the physical body as per the ancient wisdom, because for Ayurveda and yoga to work we can't afford to look upon our physical bodies the way modern science does. Let me now introduce you to the three humours or doshas as they are called – the most fundamental aspect of Ayurveda.

The Three Physical Humours

A few years ago, we were running clinical trials with a certain Ayurvedic drug formulation. This drug was a plant-based immunogen; it was supposed to boost the immune system. Two female patients reported side effects. They were in their early thirties, of similar weight, the same marital status, and with a similar lifestyle. One of them said the drug caused diarrhoea, while the other one reported constipation. While these reactions were possible, they were unusual and entirely unexpected.

We examined their eating habits. There were no anomalies. They ate moderately and healthily. In fact, they ate almost identical foods. Most notable was their regular consumption of buttermilk. We zeroed in on buttermilk. The combination of buttermilk and our drug was causing diarrhoea in one patient and constipation in the other.

Another drug was preventing hair loss in one set of patients, while the same drug had no such effect on a different set of patients. Even more intriguingly, it caused hair loss in a number of subjects.

Why were the same drugs acting differently on similar

people? Why did buttermilk cause diarrhoea in one patient and constipation in the other? Why was a drug that was supposed to strengthen hair, trigger hair loss in some patients?

One of the most outstanding aspects of Ayurveda is its teaching that nothing is absolute. The utility, value and effect of anything is relative. Hence, the efficacy of its healing is dependent on the receiver, the time and the environment. It is this profound understanding that makes Ayurveda a complete science.

Food that may be good for you could be catastrophic for another person. You may feel healthiest during the spring season, whereas another person may have the most allergies during the same period. Your medicine could well be the poison for another person.

Charaka, and other sage-physicians of his time, understood that the unique constitution of an individual was the decisive factor in how he responded to the consumption of food and medicine. One's constitution determined how one would respond to the external environment. They classified elements of the constitution with three humours: vata, pitta and kapha. The basis of Ayurveda is the understanding and application of the three humours. The sage-physicians also labelled the constitution of each individual based on the dominance of a humour or humours in his body. So, a person could be vata, pitta or kapha, or a combination of these. In this chapter, I'll elucidate the three humours, and in the next one I'll focus on the physical constitution of a person based on them.

Literally, vata means wind, pitta means bile, and kapha means mucous. These are not the complete meanings, though. Vata, pitta and kapha are not merely three physical humours; they are also three forms of energy. Vata is kinetic energy, pitta is magnetic energy and kapha is potential energy. The three humours are forever keeping your body cells in motion and your mind engaged. Vata refers to the movement of energy in your body. It controls the flow of chyle, blood, excretions and more.

Pitta, in modern terms, is metabolism. Your body has four types of digestive fires (covered later in this book). Pitta is the collective vitality of those four fires. Pitta is also the primary force behind the functioning of enzymes. Internal secretions from all glands are handled by pitta. Your body has a process of excretion at every level, from the cellular to the more prominent. Kapha is the force that is responsible for all excretion, be that perspiration, defecation, urination, ejaculation, or discharges from other bodily orifices such as ears, nostrils and eyes.

The three humours are called dosha in Sanskrit. Literally, the word dosha means fault or inconvenience. It also means alteration and morbidity. The sage-physicians carefully chose the word dosha for the three humours, because when the humours are in equilibrium, your body is healthy and normal. When one or more of the humours go out of balance, the body loses its equilibrium. The same humours become the originators of ailments. Hence the word dosha: the fault, the culprit. It is impossible for a body to be diseased when the doshas are balanced. It is only when any one of these is vitiated does a disease sprout in the body.

Equilibrium or imbalance between the doshas dictates your physical health or lack of it. Irrespective of whether a patient has a common cold or colon cancer, the cause and the cure lies in the balancing of the three humours. Complete healing, however, is not just about the three humours. The three physical humours operate in conjunction with the three mental humours. I will cover that later in this book. In the English language, no matter how long, complicated or difficult a word may be, it cannot exist outside the alphabet; it must consist of its vowels and consonants. Similarly, regardless of the stage, gravity and nature of a disease, it can only relate to the three causative humours.

Dominance of a dosha can lead to a physical disorder corresponding to its own nature. There are seven core properties of each dosha. See the table below:

The Three Doshas and Their Properties

Vata	*Pitta*	*Kapha*
Dry	Smooth	Oily
Cold	Hot	Cold
Light	Buoyant	Heavy
Subtle	Fluidal	Viscid
Kinetic	Acidic	Voluminous
Sublime	Mobile	Stable
Rough	Pungent	Sweet

An interesting question is: 'What do these properties mean?' More to the point, 'What do they mean to you?' In fact, in the ancient Ayurvedic text – *Charaka Samhita*, Charaka did not define these properties in isolation. In each of the verses specifying the characteristics of the doshas, the subsequent line says if you were to consume substances that are opposite to the properties of the dosha, it will immediately bring relief to the disorder caused by the dosha. For example, vitiated pitta can cause indigestion. If you look at the properties of pitta, it is hot, acidic, pungent and so on. Now, if you consume something that is cold and alkaline, you will get almost instant relief from indigestion.

The doshas are entirely dependent on the five great elements. As long as you have a body, the five elements will be operative and active. The doshas assume a physical form when they are transformed into organic excretions due to pathogenic or pathological factors. Vata, as air, may turn into intestinal gas; pitta, bile, may result in indigestion. Together they may lead to heartburn or acid reflux. Kapha, phlegm, may turn into mucus. It could easily be more severe in the form of residual fat clogging the vital arteries.

Your body is at the peak of its health when the doshas are in equilibrium. In some people, one dosha dominates. In fact, one dosha is almost always more active than the others. When any one dosha is vitiated, a corresponding disease manifests in the body. In some cases, however, all three doshas may be vitiated. Such a condition is called sannipata. Sanna means depressed, languid and weak, and pata means descent or death. Sannipata means the condition is severe and requires immediate attention. If the patient is not treated, the disorder can lead to an incurable chronic disease or even death.

Let me elaborate on each of the three doshas.

VATA

Vata is made up of the elements of air and ether. It is the force behind all motion in your body. Vata is cold, light and motive. It flows in the form of the ten energies controlling all kinetic aspects of your body. When vata is balanced, your speech, your gait, your glances and the movements of your limbs are all composed, minimal and graceful. When it is vitiated, it leads to erratic or excessive movements. Do you know people who move their hands too much while talking? One of the reasons for this could be imbalanced vata in their bodies.

There are six flows in your body. They are air flow, blood flow, lymph flow, gastrointestinal flow, urine flow and energy flow. Mental and physical exertion directly impact your energy flow. Further, other people's energy and the external environment can also impact your energy flow.

For example, imagine yourself in a dark room. You light a blue bulb and the whole room is now illuminated with soft blue light. Then you burn sandalwood incense. The room has a certain ambience and fragrance now. Presently, someone comes along and lights a bigger white bulb. The ambience changes immediately. Another person comes and burns strong jasmine incense. The room is the same: your bulb is just as well lit, the sandalwood scent is still in the air – but they are no longer serving their purpose. A brighter bulb and a stronger scent has veiled them.

Ayurvedic, yogic and tantric texts place great importance on energy flow. The six types of flow in your body are controlled by vata. When vata gets vitiated, diseases that are linked to the six flows manifest themselves in the human body. The patient thinks he has a gas problem, or flatulence, so he may take a pill to curb this. That is not the problem, though. It is merely the symptom. In this case vata is vitiated, so it is vata that needs to be treated.

Imagine a very large piece of barren land; a few million hectares. You are in the middle of that land. There is no water, there are no trees and no cattle. Now visualize a breeze blowing. But wait – what is your mind to see and feel? If you think of a sunny day, that breeze will feel hot and arid. On a rainy day, it'll feel colder and moist. In the same manner – and as *Sharangadhara Samhita*, a classical Ayurvedic text, states most brilliantly – 'Inert is pitta, inert is kapha, inert are the mala (residue) and dhatus. Like clouds, they go wherever they are carried by the vayu (vata or wind).'

Therefore, unless pitta or kapha is already vitiated, an imbalanced vata does no damage. If pitta is disturbed and vata gets vitiated, it will lead to gas. If vata does not get vitiated, imbalance of pitta will simply lead to indigestion or acidity. A range of symptoms, from simple twitching of the eye to permanent instability of the mind, are attributable to vata. Vata can manifest strongly and quickly. It may easily turn a small ailment into a fatal threat, just like a gust of wind can transform a small flame into a bushfire. Vata is called rogaraja, the king of all diseases.

PITTA

The primary characteristic of pitta is heat. It is chiefly made up of the fire element; its secondary element is water. Pitta is hot, acidic and pungent. It is responsible for the production of enzymes and hormones. All glands in the body secrete on account of pitta. In modern medical science, pitta represents metabolism in its entirety. The two chief aspects of metabolism – anabolism (synthesis of complex substances and storage of energy) and catabolism (breakdown of complex substances and release of energy) – are directly governed by the force of pitta. It is the bilious humour. While the three humours play an equally important role in the genesis and sustenance of a person, pitta is easily the most significant of the three, for it is the metabolic force. One's very life depends on the quality of their metabolism.

Pitta is the energy that creates and controls digestion. Along with vata, it is responsible for maintaining the body temperature. Heat in the human body exists in the form of fluids. Pitta generates the heat and vata transports it to the rest of the body. In that transportation, due to friction, vata also generates body heat.

Pitta is the transformative principle, not just for the physical body but for the psychical body as well. The processing in your brain depends on neurotransmitters. A neurotransmitter is a neurochemical substance, a type of enzyme. Thinking, contemplation and concentration are simply enzymes working in your brain. It is for this reason that meditation has a direct influence on the various functions of the brain. Modern science verifies that meditation is particularly useful in tackling mood swings, premenstrual symptoms and menopausal transition.

Given time, a cut or a wound dries up; it seems to heal on its own. This healing is predominantly due to pitta. Homeostasis – the ability of your body to maintain internal constancy and equilibrium by coordinated work of multiple complex biological agents operating in the autonomic nervous system – is a direct function of pitta.

Sometimes you shiver when you urinate, especially if it's cold. That's because your body was maintaining a certain temperature prior to urination. Hot urine in the bladder contributed to the maintenance of this temperature. And now, with urination emptying the bladder, you lose heat; your brain recognizes even the slightest drop in temperature. Consequently, the brain sends a signal, vata rushes through the sympathetic nervous system to produce that shiver, so pitta may again be brought to perfect balance. You don't shiver while voiding your bowel because pitta has enough time to restore its balance.

Any transformation occurring in your body or mind is due to pitta. Such transformation could be the breaking down of food into various nutrients ready for processing by your body, or it could be thoughts transforming into actions and goals. Without pitta, none of this is possible. When pitta is vitiated, it makes the person angry and aggressive. If vata is the kinetic energy, pitta is magnetism. It works closely with both vata and kapha for the efficient and smooth working of the complex machinery called the body.

Digestion, appetite, skin, vision, lustre and physical strength are greatly affected by pitta. Balanced pitta gives a person smooth and glowing complexion, clarity of thought, sharp intellect, perfect digestion and good vision. When imbalanced, it affects all of the above. Inflammation, swelling, discharge, itching, and perspiration are signs of vitiated pitta. Abnormal functioning of the brain and many mental disorders are also attributed to imbalanced pitta.

KAPHA

Kapha is made up from the earth and water elements. It is what holds your body together. Heavy, cold, soft and slimy, kapha represents potential energy. It is the third humour, phlegm. It is the framework, if you will. Like the other two doshas, when it is vitiated, it leaves a residue behind. In the case of kapha, such residue could be mucous, excess saliva, plaque, certain infections, stupor and lassitude.

Kapha controls vital aspects of the human body. In fact, it governs the overall structure of the body. Body growth, weight, joints, lungs, the seven dhatus, lubrication of joints, suppleness of muscles, and smoothness of internal organs are controlled by kapha. The immune system is greatly influenced by the balance of kapha in the body. Allergens are quick to attack the patient with vitiated pitta and kapha.

Kapha represents smooth skin, beautiful large eyes and silky and luxuriant hair. Its basic nature is stable. This means that when kapha is vitiated, allergies won't go away easily. The same goes for mental conditions too. Imbalanced kapha can lead one into a prolonged state of depression. The patient gains weight rather quickly. Unlike vata, kapha disorders can't be fixed overnight. If you have gas, you may drink a decoction or pop a pill and you may feel better within minutes. The same can't be said for bronchial congestion.

In short, your body frame, the strength of your joints, the type of your skin, your immune system, your mental stability, your basic nature, your complexion and many other permanent attributes of your body, are governed by kapha. Heaviness is the chief feature of kapha. When you feel heaviness in the body or mind, almost certainly it means kapha is vitiated. When you can't get up in the morning, even after a good night's sleep, it could be due to an imbalance between your kapha and vata.

Snoring is attributed to kapha. Those who snore are likely to have other disorders caused by kapha, including mucus, chest congestion and obesity, however slight. They may even be asthmatic. Kapha grants emotional and mental stability. If pitta is the solar channel in your body, kapha is the lunar channel. It helps you to go to sleep: its properties can pacify physical, mental and emotional aggression, bringing you to a state of calm and equilibrium. It is with kapha's cooperation that your body cells are repaired and healed when you rest and sleep.

The three humours determine the fundamental constitution of an individual. Each person is born with a certain constitution. It is rare for an individual to be an absolute vata, pitta or kapha. More often than not, most people have a mixed constitution. While you can't change your inherent constitution, you can modify your eating habits and your lifestyle to best suit your constitution. This is the easiest way of remaining physically and mentally healthy. Ayurveda details the method of ascertaining your constitution based on several factors.

Your Physical Constitution

Have you ever wondered why a diet programme can work splendidly for some and not at all for others? Why do some people get sick during certain seasons while others don't? Why do some get tipsy after just one drink while others can guzzle down bottles of hard liquor and still remain relatively sober? Why do some feel motion sickness even during a short trip, whereas others can travel for hours at a stretch and not feel a thing? Why do some get tired after half an hour of physical work, whereas others seem to be endowed with an inexhaustible store of energy?

Every one of us is born with a certain constitution. It determines how we accept, process and absorb the food we eat. It influences how we respond to the environment around us. The term used in Ayurveda to describe an individual's constitution is called prakriti. It means our genetic disposition, our inherent nature. This is most interesting, because the term for nature is also prakriti.

We are a part of nature. Our nature is an extract of nature itself. This is not a metaphorical statement but the firm truth. For the foods we eat, the water we drink, the air we breathe – all these were outside us once; they were in nature. Once we consume them, they are within us. They become us. We are made from them. It is, therefore, important to understand your own prakriti, constitution, so that you may know what will suit you from prakriti, nature.

The dosha you are born with is your constitution. Some have a predominance of vata, some pitta and some kapha. Many have a combination of two of these, and a rare few have the perfect balance between the three doshas. The basis of all remedies and treatments in Ayurveda is your constitution. Once you understand whether you are a vata, pitta, or kapha, or a specific combination of these, you will know what foods are good for you and which ones cause you the most damage. You will know during which seasons your immune system is the best and when it is the weakest. You can gain weight, you can lose weight; you can even cure most chronic ailments. In fact, you can enjoy near-perfect health if you get a grip on how nature responds to *your* nature.

WHAT DETERMINES YOUR CONSTITUTION

Before you ascertain which dosha you are, it will help to know the basis of your constitution. Doshas are divided into two categories: prakriti and vikriti. Prakriti is your permanent constitution. For example, if you are born fair-coloured or with a large frame, that is how you will be for the rest of your life. You cannot change your fundamental constitution. If your eyes are large, for example, that's how they will remain. Prakriti refers to one's permanent attributes. Vikriti refers to the present state of humours in your body. It alludes to fleeting ailments, seasonal mood swings and transient changes in your temperament. It is a pathological manifestation; it is symptomatic and it is temporary.

Your prakriti is not something you acquire after you are born; it is sealed in the womb, at the time you are conceived. For example, a mother who has given birth to three children would, in all likelihood, have had different issues in each pregnancy. The fetus during one pregnancy might have kicked a lot more than the others. Another baby in the womb might have been more sensitive to what the mother ate. Yet another might have been more stable than the others. The constitution is determined the moment an egg joins the sperm. It is fully manifested and mature by the time the child is delivered. This is the reason why one infant may have allergies and other constitutional disorders, whereas his sibling may be perfectly healthy. They may even be twins; even identical twins, for that matter.

There are many determinant factors that make you who you are. Your own prakriti is dependent on the constitution of the sperm and the egg, meaning your parents' constitution. The time and season during the conception play a big part in affecting your prakriti. Vedic and tantric texts lay out elaborate methods to ensure a healthy conception. The physical, mental and emotional health of the parents at the time of conception will have a telling impact on the health and temperament of the child. Further, Vedic texts strictly prohibit having sexual intercourse during the day. Both vata and pitta are aggravated from sunrise till sunset. A child conceived during the day is likely to be more aggressive and impulsive. An excess of vata leads to indecisiveness.

The physical and emotional health of the expectant mother is also a critical factor for determining prakriti.

The age and health of the uterus where the embryo lives for nine months plays an important role in this too. A late pregnancy means a weaker home for the fetus. Children of older mothers may be geniuses, but they tend to be physically weaker and more prone to allergies than their older siblings. Stress or depression for the mother during pregnancy can cause anything from simple allergies to more serious behavioural disorders in the child. In a nutshell, we have practically no control over our constitution.

EVALUATING YOUR DOSHA

There are seven possible constitutions. They are: vata, pitta, kapha, vata-pitta, pitta-kapha, vata-kapha and vata-pitta-kapha. There are specific physical and mental traits for each dosha. Simply see the ones that fit you, contemplate over it and you will know your prakriti. As I mentioned earlier, it is perfectly normal that your attributes are, for instance, vata in some and pitta or kapha in others. Very few people are absolute vatas, pittas or kaphas. Most of us are a combination of these.

PHYSICAL ATTRIBUTES

Body Frame

Vatas are thin and slender. That does not mean they lack strength or stamina. In their lean frames, they can be just as energetic as the other two doshas. Their gait is swift, and they often have long arms or long legs. They are not broad chested and tend to have a squarish body structure with small shoulders and narrow hips. Their bones are light.

Pittas have medium body frames but very symmetrical bodies. Their limbs are in proportion to the rest of their bodies. Pittas can be quite tall, but they are still well endowed with muscle. They make good fashion models. They are full of energy, but not as agile as vatas. Pitta women tend to have a natural hourglass body shape and men a natural V-shape.

Kaphas have the largest frame of the three. They have stout bodies and their build is stocky; their bones are heavy and they walk slowly. They have excellent physical strength and stamina. Many kaphas with a composite of vata make excellent athletes in sports such as rugby, boxing, weightlifting, etc.

Joints and Muscles

Vatas have prominent, sometimes protruding joints, which tend to crack easily. Do some squats: if you hear crackles in your knees, it may well mean you are a vata. Those crackles could also be due to stiffness in the body, though. Be sure to differentiate between them. Vatas' muscles are slender and have almost no fat – just flesh.

Pittas have reasonably strong joints, which are loose, well shaped and flexible. Even though their joints are good, they can develop arthritis in the later years of their life due to their pitta nature. Their muscles are well built but supple. Their muscle mass is not as lean as the vatas, but pittas have the best muscular structure from the perspective of fitness and strength.

Kaphas have large joints like their body frame. Their joints are well padded and strong, though. When standing, they can feel tiredness in their ankles very quickly, mostly because the weight of their large body frame is on their feet. This is true even if they are not overweight. This can often lead to some swelling around the ankles. Their muscles are not as lean or supple as the other two types.

Body Temperature

Vatas prefer summers. They are most productive and comfortable in warm environments. For most of the year, their hands and feet are cold. They are very sensitive towards any changes in the temperature, and their body reacts to such variations quickly.

Pittas are usually warm. They love winters and cold climates. They are uncomfortable in hot weather. They are not as bothered in changing seasons or summers as vatas are in winter. Heat tires them out quickly, however. They have the greatest physical stamina when mercury is on the lower side.

Kaphas are comfortable for most of the year, but they prefer summer and spring. Like vatas, they don't like cold days. Additionally, they feel depressed on wet days. During winters and rains, they feel low on energy and stamina.

Various seasonal affective disorders (SAD) like winter depression, winter blues or seasonal depression affect vatas and kaphas more than pittas, as people with the two former doshas experience depressive symptoms in the winter.

Body Weight

Vatas are generally underweight. If they are not underweight, they are certainly on the lighter side. They can be so excited about their passions that they may even forget to eat. Vatas have no problem with skipping meals, and they have a tendency to lose weight.

Pittas are of normal weight usually; they are just right according to their body frame. Of the three, it is the easiest for pittas to gain or lose weight. Any effects of exercise and diet shows on their body in a matter of days.

Kaphas are normally on the heavier side of the spectrum. Relative to their build, they tend to be overweight. They gain weight easily and have great difficulty in losing it. A kapha may have the strictest diet plan, yet results come slowly for him. In fact, losing weight is one of the most difficult things for kaphas.

Hair

Vatas commonly have dry hair; they get split ends easily. Their hair tends to be frizzy and breaks easily. They generally don't become bald like pittas, but they do need to take greater care of their hair. Their hair tangles easily.

Pittas mostly have extremely fine but thin hair. Their hair is long and straight and never really jet black. They tend towards blonde or red in Caucasian people and light black in Asian and African cultures. Their hair usually greys at earlier an age than vatas and kaphas. Pitta males are inclined to be bald towards the later years of their lives.

Kaphas frequently have thick and wavy hair. Their hair is oily and tends to be on the darker side. The colour of one's hair, however, is a factor almost entirely dependent on one's race. So, a Caucasian man or a woman with blonde hair could be as much a kapha as an Indian with jet black hair.

Forehead

Vatas usually have small foreheads and forward hairlines, making their foreheads look even smaller. They tend to have permanent frown marks as they age. Generally, when they raise their eyebrows, three lines appear on their forehead.

Pittas commonly have medium-sized foreheads, with wrinkles and lines in no specific pattern during the later years of their lives. Their foreheads tend to be plainer, with no frown lines or only light frown lines.

Kaphas have the largest foreheads of the three. Their foreheads are lustrous and radiant. There are usually no signs of any wrinkles there till much later in their lives.

Eyes

Vatas have small and active eyes; their eyes may even be sunken. They blink a lot and rarely settle their gaze on anything beyond a few seconds. Their eyebrows are generally smaller and frugal. Their eyelashes are of normal thickness and length.

Pittas have charismatic eyes. Their eyelashes are fine and thin. Their eyebrows are stately but not as hairy as a kapha's. Pittas have a penetrating gaze and their eyes have an artistic look.

Kaphas have large, soft and smooth eyes. There is a certain stillness and warmth in their gaze. The whites of their eyes are extremely white and prominent. Their eyebrows and eyelashes are thick and luxuriant.

Lips and Teeth

Vatas have thin lips which get dry and chapped easily. Their teeth can be somewhat uneven and may require constant care and attention.

Pittas have medium-sized soft lips. Their upper lip is slightly darker than the lower one. Their teeth are medium sized and are generally well shaped. Pittas need to take proper care of their teeth, as they tend to suffer from cavities more than both vatas and kaphas.

Kaphas have large and smooth lips. They have a slight natural pout, heightening their sex appeal. Their teeth are generally well formed and aligned and require the least care of the three types.

Skin and Complexion

While analysing your complexion, it is important to factor in your race. The darkest Caucasian is going to be several shades lighter than the lightest West African, for example.

Vatas' skin is dry and somewhat rough. They need to moisturize it properly during the dry and cold seasons to protect it from wrinkling and cracking. Their skin is thin; one can see the veins running beneath it. Their complexion is on the darker side and their skin feels cold.

Pittas have soft and smooth skin. Wrinkles don't form as easily on them as vatas. Their complexion is more on the fair side, but it tends to be wheatish or yellowish. Fair-coloured pittas suffer from skin rashes and sunburn more easily than others.

Kaphas have thick and smooth skin. Their skin is oily, and wrinkles don't appear until late in their lives. Their skin can look cold and pale. Their complexion tends to be fair and bright. Minimal skincare does it for them.

Hands and Nails

Vatas have long and slender hands. Their hands look creative and artistic; they make good surgeons and painters. The palms are somewhat dry and slightly rough. Their fingers are longer than their palms, with thin nails which crack easily.

Pittas too have somewhat long hands, but they are proportionate to the size of their bodies. Pittas make good pianists and musicians. Their fingers are slender but somewhat squarish. Their palms are slightly larger than their fingers, and their nails are square, beautiful, pink and soft.

Kaphas have short and stocky, but strong hands. Their palms and fingers are of the same length. Their nails are short and thick. With their symmetrical hands, their nails look somewhat wide and whitish.

Voice and Speech

Vatas have low voices, which may sound almost as if they are projected merely from the throat. Their voices, if projected from the chest, are deeper. They can be very talkative, speaking quickly and jumping from one topic to another.

Pittas have nicely projected voices which sound slightly nasal. They don't talk as much as vatas but can argue at great length. Their speech can often have a magnetic pull, in the sense that they sound sincere and trustworthy.

Kaphas have deep voices. They speak slowly and can remain silent for long periods. Their talking sounds like a series of prepared speeches. There are no random or redundant words: they speak with conviction, and only after thinking through what they are going to say.

Perspiration

Vatas rarely perspire. Only if they are doing heavy physical exercise do they sweat. They may sit on the beach on a sunny day without any perspiration. Their sweat is light and stays on the body. They usually have minimal body odour.

Pittas tend to sweat profusely. Small temperature variations can make them sweat. They sweat evenly on their entire body. Their body odour is not as strong as kaphas.

Kaphas perspire moderately. Their body uses sweat as a way of keeping them healthy. They tend to perspire more in certain areas of their body, notably under their arms. Their body exudes an odour stronger than both vatas and pittas.

Appetite and Digestion

Vatas have good appetites. They need their proper breakfast in the morning or they may experience headaches or heaviness in the head. Vatas have sensitive stomachs. If they eat more than what they generally do, they experience pain in their stomach or even indigestion. High-protein foods or spicy meals can upset their stomachs in no time. They are generally lactose-intolerant. Their digestion depends on the food they have just eaten.

Pittas have good appetites and phenomenal digestion. They eat at a moderate speed – not as quickly as vatas do. If they have to skip a meal, they feel irritated and unsettled. They need their three daily meals. The portion of the meals may be small, but pittas need to eat something at regular intervals. At the most, they can skip the first meal of the morning without experiencing a headache or feeling low on energy.

Kaphas have decent appetites. They are not driven by their appetites, though; they are driven by their routines. They are steady eaters. They eat slowly and they digest slowly. They can easily skip meals or fast without the slightest discomfort. They can be bulimic. Due to slow digestion and metabolism, their bodies learn to utilize internal energy stores. As a result, dietary irregularities can make them more prone to diabetes.

Sleep Pattern

Vatas are light sleepers; they can wake at the slightest of noises. They must have their required sleep. If it gets disrupted, or if they sleep less than they should in a night, they need to make up for the lost sleep within the next day or they become fidgety and irritated. They find it hard to change their sleep patterns. It takes them the longest of the doshas to get over jet lag, for example.

Pittas are moderate sleepers. They sleep lightly but soundly. Of the three doshas, pittas require the least amount of sleep to feel refreshed and recharged. They like to get out of bed as soon as they wake up and get on with their daily routine. They sometimes wake up in the middle of their sleep to drink water. They enjoy drinking water immediately after getting up. It soothes their body.

Kaphas are sound sleepers, and they can sleep for very long periods. They can easily sleep for eight to ten hours and then go back to sleep just a few hours later. They are in no rush when the morning comes. They like to lie in their beds and relax for a while before getting up to the day.

Sex Drive

Vatas have a good sexual appetite and do a lot of cerebral sex. They can do the full act in their brain. They are aroused very quickly, they become passionate just as rapidly, they get to the climax even quicker and feel exhausted afterwards. Vatas like to nap after the act. They remain sexually active till late in their lives. Their reproductive fluids are somewhat thin and flow easily.

Pittas are easily aroused and very passionate. They are more romantic than vatas but less enduring than kaphas.

Pittas are average performers. They feel hungry after the act. Their body temperature rises quickly and they sweat more than vatas and kaphas during intercourse. Unlike vatas, who have no time for foreplay, pittas care about their partners. It is not just sex but an act of love for a pitta.

Kaphas take their time to be aroused and are the most enduring of the three. Unlike vatas and pittas, for them the quality matters more than the frequency. Their virility (or fertility) is excellent. Just like with their meals, they can skip intercourse without distress, but ultimately they must have it – they can fast but cannot abstain. Kaphas may feel the urge to eat something sweet after the act.

Seasonal Allergies

When allergens are running riot during the change of seasons, vatas tend to get dry eyes. Their noses remain mostly blocked during the allergy season. There is very little discharge of mucus. They may experience chest congestion, but they get well soon enough.

If struck with hay fever, pittas get red eyes. While a vata's nose is blocked, a pitta gets a runny nose. Pittas can suffer from chest congestion, but their coughs are mostly dry. They may also experience some difficulty in breathing. It has often been observed that pittas tend to fall sick twice during the same season.

Kaphas get watery eyes when suffering from hay fever. Their noses are blocked with thick mucus and they experience the worst congestion of the chest among people of the three dosha types. Phlegm formation is the greatest in kaphas during the change of seasons.

Menstruation

Ayurveda regards menstruation as a cleansing and recharging process. The ancient texts state that the menstrual cycle is a vital indicator of a woman's health. Ideally, a woman should rest during her period, because her body is undergoing a change at this time and is under strain. Every month, nature prepares a woman for conception. It readies the womb for childbearing. During the proliferative phase, kapha, with its lubricating and stabilizing properties, prepares the uterine lining (endometrium) to grow. It nurtures and nourishes it. This is the period between cessation of flow and ovulation. If there is no union of an egg and a sperm during this period, pitta comes into play. This is the secretory phase, starting from ovulation till the period. Pitta being the dominant dosha during this phase, the basal temperature of a woman's body tends to rise. After pitta, vata dominates, and with descending energy rids the body of menstrual blood.

Vatas experience anxiety, mood swings, sleep disruption and other symptoms, such as pain in the lower back and cramps in the lower abdomen, before menstruation. Their periods are somewhat irregular and scanty; their menstrual blood is dark in colour and can be clotted. Constipation is common at this time for vatas.

Premenstrual symptoms for pittas include tenderness in the breasts, hot flushes and irritability; skin rashes and headaches are also common. Their menstrual blood is bright red and warm. Periods for pittas tend to last longer than vatas. They can experience cramps too, but not as severe as those suffered by vatas. Some pittas experience a burning sensation while urinating at this time.

Kaphas may experience bloating, water retention, and swollen and tender breasts. Their periods are not painful like those of the vatas and pittas. They may still have heavy periods though, and the blood often contains a white discharge. Kaphas experience lethargy and torpor during their periods; their metabolic processes slow down and they feel a general heaviness.

MENTAL ATTRIBUTES

Vatas are lively and bubbly people. They are enthusiastic and are keen to try new things. And they don't mind changing their opinions as they gain new information or insight. Vatas are usually extroverts. Just like the wind that's never stable, their beliefs change quickly. It doesn't take them long to form new radical beliefs. Vatas get worried and anxious quickly. But they get over their worries just as swiftly. They are quick to grasp new concepts, but their memory retention is not as good as pittas or kaphas. Vatas are quite adventurous in nature and love to spend time outdoors. They are quick-acting, accommodating and adaptable by nature. They dream a lot during their sleep but often forget their dreams.

Pittas are generally more 'head driven' than vatas. Purposeful, and at times intense, they make great leaders. They are persuasive and good at debating. Pittas can be quite aggressive and get irritated rather easily under stress. They can be irritating too at the same time. They have very good concentration and can be quite engaging. Pittas are okay with the outdoors as long as it doesn't involve rigorous activities; they enjoy more intellectual adventures. Their memories are sharp and headspaces quite clear. Possessing critical and penetrating minds, pittas are outcome-driven and goal-oriented. They dream often too, but mostly their dreams feature battles and fights or, at least, some form of violence. Pittas are somewhat impulsive; anger is their primary shortcoming. Generally, however, they have a warm nature.

Kaphas are the most stable of the dosha types. Slow, steady, easy-going and accepting, they are great supporters and loyal followers too. They are mostly introverts and become withdrawn under stress. Kaphas are happy to engage in indoor activities; outdoors and adventures are not their thing. They are slow to learn but have elephant-like memories. Their actions are thought out and rarely impulsive; they have strong preferences and don't make visceral decisions. Kaphas take their time in forming opinions but stick to them for the rest of their lives. They are generally calm and stable and can be quite lazy too. Kaphas don't dream very often but when they do, their dreams are mostly romantic.

DUAL CONSTITUTION

As I said before, it is rare for a person to be an absolute vata, pitta or kapha. Usually, people have a mixture of the doshas. If you assess yourself deeply, however, one dosha should be more dominant than the other two. The better you analyse yourself, the quicker and better you can heal yourself, because the success of all remedies, herbs and treatments in Ayurveda is dependent on how accurately your constitution is determined.

Your dosha and your prakriti represent how your genetic make-up affects your physical and mental well-being. This is only one side of the coin. Just like the three physical humours, there are also three mental humours.

When stressed, why do some people eat a lot, while many others lose their appetite altogether? Why do some get irritated easily, while many remain unaffected under the most annoying circumstances? Why do some people suffer from addictions while many don't? Why do some gain, and others lose, weight during depression? What determines these traits? What affects our mental state and why are we the way we are? Yogic texts state that just as doshas set our physical traits, our mental humours create a genetic mental disposition.

Your Mental Constitution

Omar, in his late forties, was a senior executive in a multi-billion-dollar telecommunications company. He had been happily married for twenty-one years and had a son and a daughter, both in their teens. He worked out at the gym and ate organic foods. He was in control of his professional life. The whole world, including his wife, saw Omar as a successful and happy man. He brought presents for his wife, he took his family out to dinner, they would vacation in a new country for two weeks every year. He managed his personal and professional relationships well. All in all, you couldn't possibly think that he had any problem.

Omar was healthy until recently when, out of the blue, he had three severe episodes of anxiety attacks with heart palpitations, within two weeks. He confided in me, saying that he was torn from the inside and lived in a constant state of fear and helplessness. He thought God was punishing him, because he had been sleeping with other women for years. He had started it in the fourth year of his marriage, when his wife was pregnant with their first child, seventeen years ago, he said.

Omar told me: 'I love my wife to bits. She's the perfect wife. I can't imagine living without her and I love my children. I don't want to wreck my family and my life, but I'm addicted, Swami. I'm addicted to sex. A million times I've promised myself that I will not do this to my wife, but a million times I've broken my own promise. I live with this constant guilt. I don't want to do this but I can't help it. I have tried curbing it, I've tried distracting myself, but nothing works. I know my wife will leave me if she ever finds out.

'When I look at her, I feel terrible for being disloyal to her for so long. I buy her gifts, I take her on vacations, I donate to charities, I pray, I do everything to somehow make me light, but it all fails. My past haunts me and the present tortures me. Sometimes in the middle of a meeting, and sometimes while on the treadmill, sometimes in bed, other times while reading, sometimes while watching a movie, I get these thoughts that really worry me. Even if I stop now, what will happen if something from the past springs up? I want to change, Swami. I'm tired of being like this. Please tell me why I am like this. What do I do? How do I fix myself? I think very soon I'm going to die of a heart attack. I can't take it any more.'

Omar broke down. I could see his helplessness.

'Omar,' I said, 'I'll ask you just two questions. If the answer is yes to both of them, I know I'll be able to help you. If not, you'll have to see a therapist.'

'Anything, Swami.'

'Was your father an aggressive man? And did your mother put up with his aggression?'

'Yes, Swami. Sometimes she answered back, but it was always a mistake because first my father would shout at her and then withdraw for days and weeks at a stretch to punish her. The atmosphere at home would be extremely tense and unbearable.'

'Okay then, Omar. I know what we need to do. I'm not a psychologist or a therapist. But I will tell you that you have to become a strict vegetarian and you have to practise a certain type of meditation. I promise you'll see the results within three months.'

Omar emailed me every two weeks with a progress report. Three months later he saw me again and said he hadn't ever felt as light, energetic, calm or happy. Meditation and a change in his diet worked for him. It's been over two years, and his sexual urges no longer drive him insane. He wanted to know how and why it worked, but more than that, he was intrigued. What did his father's aggression or mother's suffering have to do with his sexual temperament and conduct? And particularly, how did becoming a vegetarian have an impact on his sexual addiction?

It was quite simple from my perspective. Just like the three physical humours, there's a certain genetic mental disposition everyone is born with. This relates to the mental or the psychical humours. They are purity (sattva), passion (rajas) and aggression (tamas). Omar was not conceived in an act of love but lust. His father must have been aggressive at the time. Like an animal, he was simply looking for an outlet to sate his lust. His mother was unhappy in the relationship and felt betrayed, for her husband's actions had no care, no tenderness and no love. In the mixture of passion and lust, in the combination of confusion and indifference, Omar was conceived. I asked him to become a vegetarian because non-vegetarian food is tamasic in nature. Although I've seen many vegetarians with similar issues, I particularly wanted Omar to stay off anything that strengthened his genetic disposition.

He was born out of passion and aggression and, as a result, for the better part of his grown-up life, Omar experienced uncontrollable sexual urges. Aggression doesn't always mean that you yell or be feisty. Many people express it by withdrawing from others. Either way, it is tamas. Withdrawing to avoid someone is not the same as withdrawing to punish her. Tamas can express itself in the form of extreme negative emotions: anger, hatred or aggression. Omar's tamas was not in his behaviour towards his wife but in his untamed libido. Our mental humours are the primary driving force behind our habits. Whether they are eating, sleeping, sexual or social habits, behind all our reactive and impulsive actions, the subtle forces of nature are working. These are called the modes of material nature. They have the same name as the mental humours. In fact, the scriptures make no distinction between individual dispositions and the modes of material nature. They are identical because we are nature.

Ayurveda specifically documents the correlation and interdependence between one's mental and physical states. Your state of mind affects your physical health and your physical health impacts your mental state. Just as your physical body is governed by the three humours, your mind is governed by the three mental humours. The physical humours are called dosha; literally, fault, principally because they require a most careful balance. An excess in any dosha is never good for the body. Doshas must be balanced and moderated. The mental humours, on the other hand, are not called dosha but guna. Guna means quality.

Taking a cue from yogic and Vedic texts, Ayurveda recognizes that the humours of the mind cannot be absolutely bad or absolutely good. They are subjective. Aggression of the mind may be detrimental to your digestion, but if you are a soldier out on the battlefield, you need adrenaline pumping through your body: you need that aggression to fight, to survive – to do your job. Hence, the humours of the mind are known as virtues or qualities, because it's not so much about what we have as much as it is about how we use what we have.

The health of your nervous system, vitals and digestion – and the strength of your immune system – have a direct and definitive correlation with the three mental humours. Unlike the physical humours, these three humours are not permanent. They are forever fluctuating in every individual. Sometimes rajas will win over tamas, other times tamas will win over rajas, and sometimes sattva will win over both. This constant struggle between the humours is the cause of varying moods and mental states in people. Anyone in a physical body is affected by the mental humours. With mindful and righteous living, it is possible to tame the fluctuations to a great degree, directly improving your physical and mental health. Let me elucidate the three humours for you.

IGNORANCE

This is called tamas in Sanskrit. Tamas also means darkness, illusion, error and gloom. It primarily refers to a state of aggression. Nature destroys with tamas. The functions of deterioration, death, decay, disintegration and complete destruction are governed by the mode of ignorance. Anything comprising the five elements must eventually decay. This is the fate of any material entity. These entities may be living or non-living, moving or still, natural or artificial, organic or inorganic. Upon decomposition, they merge back into the five elements.

No matter how dearly or intelligently you hold on to whatever matters to you, eventually it will meet destruction; it will separate from you. The fundamental law of nature is that everything must go back to its original state. If you boil water and leave it aside, it will go back to a normal temperature. It can't remain hot forever. If you freeze it and leave it aside, it'll go back to being water. This is the law of nature. So, not only is tamas not bad, it is necessary, because it is simply the stage before restoration and rejuvenation. The destruction in tamas is illusory, because nothing is really getting destroyed. Only the forms are changing; it is merely a change of appearance – a sort of transformation.

Tamas in the human mind is the seed of aggression, negativity, hatred, depression, delusion, fear and anger. In the darkness of tamas, in that illusion, one no longer sees right from wrong. In fact, its rising and gripping ignorance justifies all wrong acts as right. Whether it's partners lying to each other, people killing each other, governments fooling their people, or countries going on a spree of territorial aggression, tamas makes it all look like a normal part of our contemporary world.

Additionally, tamas means inertia, dullness and lethargy. Ego is tamas.

PASSION

Passion is called rajas in Sanskrit. Rajas also means blood. Interestingly, rajas also means a vaporous cloud or a sphere of mist. It is this description that gives us the real insight into the nature of passions: they are impermanent and fugacious. Like a cloud of mist, they disappear as soon as they appear. This is the essence of human life.

Throughout our lives we work hard to feel good, to feel happy. But pleasures are never like the gentle stream – they come in squirts and spurts, as if happiness is teasing us. All pleasures spring from the pursuit of passion. The writer at his desk, the athlete on the field, the scientist in her lab, and the artist with her painting – they all derive a certain pleasure in pursuing their passion. Every time a passion is fulfilled, it gives us a glimpse of happiness. A neurotransmitter is fired in the brain. It feels good. This tiny experience of happiness and euphoria subsides after a while, and then we begin pursuing the passion again.

Think of someone overcome with passion and engaging in the sexual act. It disappears completely as soon as they are done. The passion is gone. Fast-moving currents in a river of urges flow into a gentle sea of calmness and equipoise. Till they come back, that is. This is the nature of passion: it's transient, it's short lived, it's temporary.

Rajas sits in the middle of the modes of ignorance and goodness, because during the arousal of passion, one may lean towards either ignorance or goodness. When one's passion is dominated by ignorance, one could easily harm the other person or even take someone's life. But when goodness dominates passion, one may even jump into the sea, risking one's life to save another person. Passion, when tamed and harnessed, brings out the extraordinary in an individual. Such a person may become an inventor, a scientist, a mathematician, a preacher, an artist, a musician, a peace worker or an administrative officer. When it is channelled, this energy bestows exceptional absorption, concentration and persistence on a person.

The fact that the word rajas also means blood signifies that every person has some passion, just as everyone has blood in their bodies. Not everyone discovers their passion, though. Each individual has certain talents and passions hidden in them; it's in their blood. It's only a matter of bringing them out. Nature creates with rajas. Therefore, in your microcosm too, creativity is a function of passion. Rajas represents transience, desire and action.

PURITY

Purity is called sattva in Sanskrit. Sattva also means goodness, light and knowledge. But most importantly, it means your innate nature; your basic fabric. Your inherent nature is pure bliss and light. Imagine you are hiding a small lamp in your hands and you walk into a dark room. As soon as you open your hands, the whole room will light up. The light in your hands has removed the darkness. But what if you walk into a lit room, hiding a bit of darkness in your closed hands? The room will not become dark when you open your hands. There'll be light all around. Because light is the dharma of nature; it is the way of nature. Similarly, our own true nature is light and bliss. If we become aware of our passions and ignorance, they automatically become feeble, because sattva is boosted with awareness.

In fact, yogic and Ayurvedic texts mention knowledge (jnana), scientific knowledge (vijnana), restraint (samyam), mindfulness (smriti) and concentration (ekagrata) as the antidote and treatment for mental afflictions caused by imbalanced mental humours. Each of these five strengthens sattva.

The sage-physician Charaka makes it clear that ignorance

and passion can be faults, and therefore may be detrimental to a person's physical and mental health, but sattva can never be harmful – no matter what. Sattva represents the quintessential mental, psychical and emotional balance. Nature sustains with sattva. If nature goes out of balance, the world will cease to exist. If rajas is pleasure and joy, then sattva is happiness and bliss.

The constant play and competition between sattva, rajas and tamas triggers changes in mood, emotion and the flow of thoughts. Tamas causes a disease, rajas treats it and sattva heals the sufferer. Sattva represents steadiness, peace, clarity and balance.

Imagine someone shouts at you aggressively, with an intent to upset you. If, then, you contemplate physically abusing or harming this person, it means tamas is strong; it is governing you. In the same situation, if you feel your aggressive emotions well up, but you do not yell at the other person, rajas has won over tamas. If, however, you don't feel any negativity or aggression; you don't feel like giving it back to the person, nor do you have to curb your reaction – in simple terms, you remain unaffected – it means that your mode of goodness, sattva, has won over both tamas and rajas.

Our mental and physical humours have an intricate relationship with the energy flow and the digestive fire in our bodies. Vedic texts list many types of fire, notably, the fire of wisdom (jnana-agni), the fire of the senses (darshana-agni), the fire of passions (kama-agni) and the fire of love (prema-agni). For our benefit or to our detriment, these are the fires that heat, transform, mould and shape us. When unchecked, they can also burn us. Most people in our world are burning in one or more of these fires – the burning to have more money, be famous, be recognized, own something, have someone, be something and do more. These fires first give us warmth, then they dry us out – and then they burn us. These mental fires arise out of fluctuations in our mental humours. They affect the fire in our body directly, impacting our health and well-being.

There are thirteen fires in the human body controlling various metabolic functions in the organs and tissues and at a cellular and molecular level. Of these, the four digestive fires are dominant; they govern the others.

THE FOUR TYPES OF DIGESTIVE FIRES

Fire does not discriminate between the good and the bad. It rejects nothing. Imagine a fireplace in a wooden cottage, well lit and heated. The embers are glowing and the wood is burning. If this fire goes out of control, it will burn the house down. The fire does not differentiate between the firewood and the wood that the house is made of. A similar lack of discrimination is a critical property of digestive fire. First, it burns the fluids in the stomach, then it burns the solids. If it does not die down, it first burns the vital bodily fluids (apa) and then the life force (prana); the person feels acidic, suffers from heartburn and becomes parched and dehydrated. Digestive fire only helps the body if it is moderated and managed.

The fire in the physical body is called jathara-agni in Ayurveda. Jathara means stomach and agni means fire. It helps every living entity digest food. The Vedas name it vaishvanara. It means universal, sacred and the sun. From the outside it may appear that our bodies are generating heat, but the view of the Vedas is far more profound than that.

The digestive fire is also called the sun, because everything we consume already has the fire of the sun in it. Grains, vegetables, roots – or, in fact, any food items – they were all nourished by the sun before they became our food. Hence, the heat was already in them. Our metabolic processes simply reclaimed the heat and passed it on to our system. Later in this book, I talk about how food can be hot or cold – not just in temperature, but in its effect on the body. For now, let me elaborate on the four types of digestive fire.

Balanced Fire

It is called sama-agni. Sama means even and balanced. A stomach with a balanced digestive fire is the sign of a healthy body. In fact, a body can only remain healthy if the digestive fire is in balance. Sama-agni means that vata, pitta and kapha are even and not vitiated at all. Food digests and assimilates properly in those endowed with balanced digestive fire. It increases the quality of the seven dhatus. It not only leads to fine physical health but perfect mental equilibrium too.

Wicked Fire

Wicked fire is called vishama-agni. When wind (vata) is vitiated and it affects your digestive fire, it is called vishama-agni. Imagine a flag planted in a place where the wind is blowing sporadically. The flag flutters whenever the wind blows and remains still otherwise. Similarly, vishama-agni alternates between increased secretion of digestive juices and then barely any secretion. The food either gets digested too quickly or too slowly. The patient may think that something is wrong with his food, but his problem is an imbalanced digestive fire. It can lead to diarrhoea, dysentery, stomach ulcers, rumbling in the stomach, flatulence and eructation.

Sharp Fire

Sharp fire is called tikshna-agni in Sanskrit. When digestive fire is imbalanced due to vitiated heat (pitta), the condition of tikshna-agni arises. The word tikshna also means acidic. This fire is particularly acidic in nature. Regardless of the type of food consumed, it digests rather quickly. A person with tikshna-agni tends to feel hungry again soon after having his meal. As soon as the food digests, his throat, mouth cavity and lips become dry. There is a burning sensation in his chest and stomach which robs his body of its strength. Tikshna-agni can cause anomalies in urine, colic, hyperacidity and vertigo. In some cases it can also lead to hepatomegaly or haematoma.

Slow Fire

Slow fire is called manda-agni. When deranged phlegm (kapha) affects the digestive fire, it becomes manda-agni. Manda means slow. A patient with manda-agni eats much less than the average person, and even then is unable to digest the smallest quantity of food. He is particularly intolerant of dairy products and feels heaviness in the abdomen and head. This is a highly unhealthy condition. The undigested food produces toxins that rise through the windpipe causing it to swell temporarily, creating breathing difficulties and other problems. This is the primary cause of asthma, bronchitis, cough, nausea and fatigue. Patients suffering from manda-agni suffer from irregular bowel movements, and they also tend to drool while sleeping due to excess salivation.

People governed by sattva generally have a balanced fire. Those with a predominance of rajas tend to have either wicked or sharp fire, depending on the state of vata in their body. Those with more tamasa have slow fire. We can either align our mental humours and fix our physical ailments, or we can change our lifestyle and soothe our mental afflictions. Neither option is mutually exclusive. Yogic scriptures advocate building a mental and moral discipline to attain perfect health. Ayurveda, on the other hand, focuses on the outward influencing the inward. It encourages an external discipline to feel happy and healthy. It demonstrates how food can transform us.

Ayurveda states that one should consume foods according to one's constitution. When we do that, our nature starts to synchronize with nature, and the foods we eat lead to better health and harmony. Each food has a certain quality that affects our well-being. Just like we have physical and mental humours, food too has something similar.

Every natural food has a living energy in it. This is the mystical aspect of our food. It is why the fermentation of grapes and the fermentation of wheat are not the same. Even if two foods have identical tastes throughout the four stages of digestion, it doesn't mean that they'll have the same effect on your mind. In the short term, they may appear to have the same effect on your body. But ultimately, it's their effect on your mind that will determine the outcome for your body.

Foods invigorate or aggravate your genetic disposition. The food you eat and the manner in which you eat it makes a great difference to your physical and mental health. No, I'm not asking you to become a vegetarian, I'm simply giving you a new perspective on food.

We Are What We Eat

Why do we consume food? Clearly, it is not just for survival. We are more evolved than that. If it were just for sustenance, half of life's struggles would disappear, because we would just eat anything at all and not be concerned with the taste and flavour. The truth is, we expect a certain fulfilment from the food we consume. It is the reason we tend to go out sometimes, or eat different cuisines or even just different food items. Each type of food offers us a slightly different experience. Our mind craves the experience that only comes from consuming certain foods. But what is it in the food that makes us feel that way?

Vedic scriptures state that across all the animate and inanimate living entities, there are 8.4 million species on our beautiful planet. These are spread across the numerous plants, mammals, worms, birds, sea life and other species. We are one of the 8.4 million species. Every living entity is born with a certain natural tendency. It's called svabhava. Sva means natural or normal, and bhava means sentiment or tendency.

The natural tendencies of a creature compel it to behave

in a certain way. A tiger may pounce, a deer may be frightened easily, a bull may charge, a cow may tolerate, a snake may rattle and a scorpion may sting. They are born with a set of natural traits. This energy of tendencies never really dies but gets transferred from one entity to another. Even plants have it. It is indestructible – every cell of your body is infused with this energy.

Some plants grow in spring, while some trees give fruits in autumn; many flourish in summer whereas some do in winter. It is their svabhava – their natural tendency. Whatever we eat, by digesting it we reclaim its energy and it becomes a part of our system. The energy of the food affects our energy. It has a significant influence on our physical, emotional and mental well-being. Everything we eat is one of the 8.4 million species and as such has certain tendencies. Those tendencies are divided into three categories, namely, purity (sattvic), passion (rajasic) and ignorance (tamasic). Yes – they are named after our three mental humours of sattva, rajas and tamas.

THE THREE TYPES OF FOOD

Anything your body digests is food. How your body processes food and how much you benefit from this processing depends on your attitude towards food, towards life, towards yourself and towards others. It depends on your mental state. When we consume food, it is not just about eating, digesting and excreting. We have, in fact, made a silent agreement with the food. We have agreed to absorb the energy from the food along with its svabhava. We are about to become the food we've just consumed.

Ayurveda and yogic texts state that the nature of our

food is inseparable from our own nature. When we eat sattvic food, it gives us inner clarity, determination and peace. Rajasic food fuels our passions, and tamasic food creates aggression and restlessness. They are named after the three mental humours, because food has a direct impact on your state of mind. For example, alcohol, coffee and tea can have an almost immediate effect on your mental state.

The ancient yogis spent a majority of their time in meditation and related practices. But they long realized two fundamental truths of our existence. First, there is little joy in living or even in meditating in the absence of good physical health, and second, the foods we consume can trigger thoughts, emotions and feelings. The yogis figured a calm mind was infinitely more powerful than a restless mind. They considered food the most important factor for a calm mind and good physical health. Upon deep contemplation, they also recognized that food could be the greatest obstacle to good health. Based on the mental humours, they expounded the classification of inherent tendencies of foods, dividing them into the three categories of sattvic, rajasic and tamasic.

Sattvic

Created from the word sattva, food full of goodness is called sattvic. The Bhagavadgita lists ten characteristics of sattvic food. Sattvic food supports the seven dhatus in our body by providing nutrition at each of the four stages of the food's processing by the body. Due to its natural tendency of light and goodness, it strengthens the body, boosts our physical health and calms the mind. Sattvic food, being inherently pure, arouses emotions of love and compassion. All living creatures eat, but we are the only ones with refined taste.

Therefore, sattvic food should be sumptuous and not too dry, because good food purifies us. Sattvic food pacifies the three doshas; nutrition is its hallmark. Further, it promotes overall well-being and ensures longevity.

Above all, sattvic food promotes mental stability and quiescence. Think of some of the vegetarian mammals in our world – cows, camels, elephants, goats, sheep, deer and giraffes. What comes to your mind when you visualize them? They all have big, compassionate eyes. They are all docile creatures. Their sight immediately arouses compassion and love in the viewer. There's a fundamental difference between carnivores and herbivores. The herbivores mostly sit with their front legs tucked in while the carnivores sit with their frontal limbs spread. Omnivores alternate between the two postures. Vedic texts regard the former posture as a sign of an inward mind that promotes stability and grace in movements. Sattvic food naturally makes you turn inward. You don't feel the urge to spread yourself.

Most wholesome food items like fresh vegetables and fruits fall into the sattvic category. The alkaline foods of our present world are synonymous with the sattvic foods of olden times. The only exception is dairy food – Ayurveda treats milk, butter and clarified butter as sattvic, whereas contemporary medical science considers it acidic. We will get to more of that in the sub-chapter 'Acidic and Alkaline Foods'.

Rajasic

Foods that arouse passion and desires are called rajasic. These foods make a person restless or too active, and have a negative effect on memory, disposition, calmness and physical health. In particular, if they are consumed even somewhat excessively or carelessly, it vitiates the three doshas. Foods that are too bitter, too hot, too spicy, too pungent, too salty, too dry or too acrid are rajasic foods. These foods are the source of suffering, the yogis say.

According to them, it is better to have a calm mind free of desires than to have a restless mind full of unfulfilled ones, because non-fulfilment of desires leads to depression and sadness. Let's take the example of Vishy, a man in his late thirties. Vishy used to live in a small and quiet house with his wife and two daughters. He worked as a supervisor in a factory and made enough money to have a basic but decent lifestyle. He was debt-free. The real-estate market crashed and the price of houses fell by more than thirty per cent. Vishy and his wife couldn't resist temptation. They sold their primary home, also at the prevailing lower market price, took out a mortgage and bought a million-dollar home, because they believed they got it thirty per cent cheaper.

Vishy's salary now proved inadequate to take care of living expenses. He started working over the weekends. The interest rate was hiked by the federal bank. Suddenly, they were struggling to make ends meet. Sometimes, they used their credit card to pay for the essentials. It began adding up and before they knew, they were twenty thousand dollars in credit card debt, even though they hadn't been on a vacation in five years.

His wife also started working and this upset their lifestyle. Both would come home stressed, and there was no time left to spend with the children and each other. Happy life as they knew had disappeared like the morning dew upon sunrise. They worked like this till their retirement to become debt-free again, and figured that in the preceding twenty-five years, they had paid three-and-a-half times their borrowing. Practically, they had worked day and night for seventeen years of their lives just to pay bank interest. Their kids had long since moved out, and the rooms in the house were now mostly empty. When they were finally free to enjoy life with their savings, they had little energy left. Years of neglect had given many ailments a permanent home in their bodies and minds.

All of this could have been avoided; it was unnecessary, in fact. If only they had dropped the thought of a million-dollar home, it would not have become a desire. They would then have not felt the urge to pursue it. But what has all this got to do with rajasic food, you may ask? Here it is: the ability to drop a thought or focus your attention elsewhere is dependent on your state of mind. A restless mind can't drop a thought; only a stable and calm mind can. Rajasic foods make you more active – they make you more restless and fuel the thoughts and consequently the desires.

Almost all seafood, spices, and most grains, beans and lentils fall in the category of rajasic food. All soft drinks and junk foods are rajasic foods.

Tamasic

There are certain foods that wreak havoc on your physical and mental health. These are called tamasic foods.. The next time you take frozen cooked food and heat it to eat, pay attention to your state of mind. I guarantee that it will leave you feeling lethargic. Cooking frozen ingredients and cooking fresh food won't give you the same feeling. The frozen food will at best be nearly as good as fresh food. But reheating food that has already been cooked turns it into tamasic food. Your stomach may be full, but the natural tendency of the food is now tamasic.

Foods that are not freshly prepared, ill-cooked, insipid, putrid and burnt are tamasic. Foods that are stale, impure and unnatural are also tamasic. These foods make us lethargic and ultimately create aggression in our minds. They confuse the digestive forces of the physical body, as our body does not know how to break down unnatural foods. They also tend to take much longer to digest, causing acidity, heartburn, reflux, stomach ulcers and irregular bowel movements. Further, they generate excessive heat in the body. As a result, tamasic foods cause imbalance in the body.

Acidic foods are mostly tamasic. All canned and processed foods these days are tamasic. All meats are tamasic, and all red meets are highly tamasic.

We no longer live on trees or in caves; we no longer hunt on a day-to-day basis – we live in air-conditioned homes, we work in heated offices, and our vehicles have climate control. There is no real reason for sticking to our primitive dietary habit of meat eating.

Doubtlessly, societies in many parts of the world have been living a certain lifestyle for thousands of years. There, people's bodies have adjusted to certain foods – and so have their minds. And someone living in Tibet or the Arctic tundra can't be expected to be a vegetarian, because there's barely any vegetation in these places to begin with. But these can't be valid excuses for the rest of us – who have better options available and who live in warmer regions – to ignore our evolving consciousness.

During certain yogic practices of mental, physical and emotional detoxification, the aspirant is asked to observe a strict diet. It is called havishya-anna. The rationale behind the diet is brilliant and ingenious. Havishya-anna means food that is fit for the gods. Literally, it means food that is fit for oblations. Your body is the temple, the altar, and deserves your utmost respect; the living god in your body is your mind. Your food is one of the greatest offerings to this god – it affects both your body and your mind.

For a certain stretch of time – generally forty days, but sometimes many months – the yogis would go on the havishya diet. The rules were simple: no grains, no beans, no lentils, no gluten and no salt. Milk, butter, clarified butter, honey and sea salt were allowed, along with fruits and vegetables. During many of my own practices, I have lived on the havishya diet multiple times over the past two decades. It has been my personal experience that it truly does bring great calmness and positive changes in your health.

OXIDATIVE DAMAGE AND TAMASIC FOODS

In Ayurveda and yogic texts, any food that is not freshly cooked or made from fresh ingredients is deemed tamasic food. As covered earlier in this chapter, such food promotes ill health. It is often the root cause of disease, because tamasic food leads to excessive free radicals in the body. Often, in olden times, people had a few leaves of tulsi (*Ocimum sanctum*) after their meal, because tulsi is rich in antioxidants. Or people consumed a pickle of lemon, mango or amlaki (*Emblica officinalis*), that was rich in vitamin C and had a healthy dose of antioxidants.

What is the connection between tamasic foods and free radicals? Modern research has proven beyond doubt that oxidation of food is one of the major causes of inflammation in the body. Inflammation is the culprit in almost all major bodily ailments. It is either the direct cause, result or a significant contributory factor in most chronic disorders, from asthma to cancer.

Oxidation is your food going rusty. Think of a piece of iron that is in a moist, wet or marshy area. It is going to rust quickly. Exactly the same thing happens with your food. When it has been cooked for a while, it gets oxidized. Cut an apple and leave it out for a few minutes and it goes brown; it gets oxidized. Squeeze a few drops of lemon on the apple you have cut, and it doesn't go brown because the vitamin C in the lemon prevents oxidation.

An ideal diet must have a portion of foods rich in antioxidants. Free radicals damage your skin, cells and arteries. They are capable of inflicting harm on your very DNA. The two chief methods of avoiding oxidative damage is by eating freshly prepared meals and ensuring an intake of foods rich in antioxidants. Lemons and most citrus fruits rich in vitamin C are an excellent source of antioxidants. Most berry fruits such as strawberries, blueberries, raspberries and cranberries are packed with antioxidants. Beans such as small red beans, red kidney beans, pinto beans and black beans have plenty of oxidants. Chlorinated water is highly oxidized and should be avoided as much as possible. You should drink good water. And yogic texts believe that deep breathing, which will flush your body with excess oxygen, also helps in balancing some of the ill effects of consuming tamasic foods.

Compare two burgers: one made at a fast-food outlet and the other one made at home. If you make a fresh burger at home, even though it is junk food, the damage to your health is going to be far less than when you eat a burger with identical ingredients at a fast-food outlet. According to Ayurveda, there are many factors other than the actual food that determine the effect of the food on your body. Such factors include; who prepares your food and under what conditions, the surrounding environment where you consume your food, your own state of mind, the freshness and quality of the ingredients, the time of consumption and the time taken to eat your food. These factors determine the nourishment (or lack of it) that you will derive from your meal.

You don't have to be a fanatic or a food freak. It's okay to indulge sometimes. An occasional cup of coffee, a glass of wine or a gratifying dessert with egg in it may all be okay. For that matter, anything is okay as long as it doesn't become a part of your routine – as long as it doesn't become a habit. If you remember that your body is paying a price for everything you consume, you are free to eat whatever you fancy.

In earlier times, people ate more and they worked more. The tiredness from their physical work allowed them to sleep well. They lived in close-knit communities – a support system that helped them stay relatively free of stress. They prepared meals made from fresh and wholesome foods; the water they drank was free of chlorine or any other chemicals. Pesticides or artificial fertilizers did not exist. It was a perfectly balanced, natural and sustainable environment.

That is all there is to good health: eat well, exercise well, sleep well and be happy. In the present day and age, some of these may be a long shot. But you can still eat wholesome foods with a grateful attitude; you can still do physical workouts; your life and living can still have a discipline; you can choose to respond to stressful situations in a more composed and calm manner; you can cut down on your television and Internet time – and consequently enjoy the unique benefits that come from good health alone. For these, there is no substitute. And it all begins with knowing what to eat and how to eat it.

Medicine Cures, Food Heals

While growing up, I was severely asthmatic. My father took me to every chest specialist and every doctor anyone recommended. He had more belief in the modern system of medicine than Ayurveda. Ultimately, when all else failed, we ended up at the clinic of an Ayurvedic doctor. In his late fifties, the doctor was soft-spoken and extremely knowledgeable. He checked my pulse, examined me compassionately and prescribed a couple of Ayurvedic medicines. At the back of the prescription, he patiently scribbled a long list of foods I was to avoid. Considering my constitution, he asked me to avoid potatoes, mangoes, too many sweets, yogurt and cold water, among a few other things.

I frowned at him because I loved mangoes. If I wasn't allowed to have sweets, of what use was human life, I thought. Yogurt was my favourite. I wasn't too fussed about potatoes. But no cold water? I felt that God had sent this doctor to ruin my life. I would always try my best to avoid visiting him, because in front of my father he would ask me if I'd been observing the restrictions on my diet. The truth was difficult and lying wasn't an option.

The truth was difficult indeed, because the truth was that if I wanted to cure myself, I had to consider food as part of my medicine. Why part? It was the medicine! This was a lesson I learned much later. The carbohydrates in the prohibited foods were causing inflammation of my airways, making it difficult for me to breathe. I was too young to realize this back then.

I kept eating the forbidden foods, and the medicines had little effect. I kept falling sick at the change of seasons. But a couple of severe asthma attacks when I was fourteen made me rethink things. I began following the dietary recommendations, and I never popped another allopathic pill for my asthma. I kept inhalers with me, just to be on the safe side, but at least no chemical was going into my stomach. Nothing was making me drowsy or tired now. I realized that food truly was my medicine.

We are what we eat. This is not philosophy but science. Think about this: you consume an apple and a little while later, once it is processed by your body, the apple has become a part of your body. You are the apple; your body is entirely made from the food you consume. Therefore, you underestimate the importance, role and medicinal value of food at your own peril.

The food you eat is consumed by the digestive fire in your body. Some foods fuel your digestive fire, some merely aid it and some extinguish it. Imagine a fire pit where a fire is blazing. If you put butter in it, it will flare up. If you stoke it with firewood, it will burn longer. If you pour water on it, it will douse the fire. According to Ayurveda, what may fuel your fire may douse another person's fire. No one food is good for everyone. It depends on your own mental and physical constitution. Food has a nature of its own. Food is not independent from health; health is not independent from food. What is nectar for your body could poison another person's body.

Therefore, most anomalies in physical health can simply be remedied by eating the right food. Not only this; if you eat the right food, the chances are that such ailments won't even emerge in your body. The more you know yourself (by identifying your physical and mental humours), the better you can judge the food you should be eating. The rule of thumb is to avoid consuming food that is not congenial to your own temperament.

Ayurveda is perhaps the only system of medicine that places an extraordinary emphasis on food. So much so that, in Ayurveda, the food a patient can eat is often prescribed just as a physician would prescribe medicine. There is a profound rationale behind this. Think about it: the amount of food we consume is far greater than the amount of medicine we may take. We may swallow some pills weighing a few grams, whereas the mass of food we consume is several hundred times greater. And ultimately, all food we ingest gets processed by the stomach and becomes part of us.

The modern system of medicine specializes in the treatment of symptoms. For example, how do painkillers work? What happens if you have a backache? The back sends a signal to the brain that something's not quite right there. The brain receives these signals and responds with a pain signal that prompts you to do something about it. If you go to a doctor with this pain, he'll give you a chemical that will first go in your stomach and then through the blood to reach the affected area. The receptors there either stop receiving the pain signals from the brain or stop sending those signals to the brain asking for help.

It's doing practically nothing for the root cause of the pain. It can't, because the physician hasn't found the root cause. If the ailment is minor, for the little while when the signal is not being sent or received, the body heals itself and you are cured. Even this doesn't sound like a bad idea. The real issue arises when the ailment is not minor. You keep taking painkillers, and eventually your brain gets used to the chemical and refuses to let it interfere with its job. No matter how much you increase the dosage, the brain will get used to it. Eventually, the painkillers will stop working. And then the physician will either change the painkiller or tell you that nothing can be done for you.

Ayurveda and yogic texts look upon this problem differently. They don't believe that all your intelligence resides in your brain. Since metabolism is occurring even at a cellular level, it is evident that each cell has a certain intelligence, almost like its own brain. Any colony of cells can form a self-healing network. This is why an ointment helps in healing a wound; it's communicating directly with the local brain. The formation of pus or the clotting of blood – the healing of the wound – are all due to the cells' local intelligence. And this brings me to the crux of the matter.

Food is your greatest medicine. You consume medicines in milligrams. What chance does twenty or two hundred milligrams of a chemical have to interact with or influence the local intelligence in the body? Compare this to one kilogram of food you may eat every day. This is ten thousand times more than one hundred milligrams. It reaches every single cell of your body. The goal of Ayurveda is to interact with the local intelligence, and it does it by way of prescribing food based on the humours and other treatments – massage, oil bath, steam, purgation, etc.

Ayurveda categorizes all foods based on their taste. Taste in Ayurveda doesn't only mean how it tastes, but how it impacts the health. For example, vata is cold and dry, so foods that are hot and rich in fat are good for the vata person. This seems contrary to the contemporary food sense, where foods with fat are avoided by most health-conscious people. This is a mistake because fat, like carbohydrates and protein, belongs to the fundamental group of nutrients. Fat is as essential as any other nutrient. This doesn't mean, however, that everyone will be okay having the same amount of fat. To help people with different constitutions, pick the right food. Ayurveda intelligently classifies food in six tastes.

THE SIX TASTES

All food is made up of the five elements and together they produce six tastes. They are sweet, sour, salty, pungent, bitter and astringent. Each food has a unique combination of the six tastes. Variations in the combination gives a food its distinctive flavour. In various permutations and combinations, the six tastes create sixty-three different flavours. Of the five elements, water is the primeval source of taste. In its own right, it is soothing, cold, light and devoid of any taste. However, it either accentuates or pacifies the inherent taste of a food. Lack of water concentrates the taste and excess of it leads to dilution of the taste. This is water's only role across the six tastes.

Further, Ayurveda states that seasons have a bearing on the taste of foods. For example, the taste of an out-of-season mango tends to be sour. Also, one of the properties of pitta is acidic. If a pitta person was to consume a sweet mango during the season, it would do him no harm, but if he consumed a sour mango, it would aggravate his acidity. The six tastes are not merely about how they taste on the tongue but how your body tastes them. Let me elaborate on this subtle but profound difference, beginning with an elucidation of the six tastes.

Sweet

Water is the primary element of this taste, known as madhura in Sanskrit. The sweetness is due to the water element. Classical tantric texts state that earth too is an element in this taste. Madhura is nourishing, delightful to the sense organs and conducive to longevity. It promotes all dhatus, strength and lustre. It allays pitta, quenches thirst and provides energy to the mind and body. It is heavy, unctuous and cold.

Madhura is good for the throat, skin and hair. With immoderate consumption, it vitiates kapha and promotes obesity, coughing, sinusitis, dyspnoea, lethargy, heaviness, constipation and difficult bowel movements or incomplete bowel evacuation. It can contribute to hardening of the arteries, thereby posing a risk of heart disease too. It dims and even deludes the appetite. In line with modern medical thought, in Ayurveda, a diabetic patient is advised to completely avoid foods with a sweet taste. Even five thousand years ago, Ayurvedic practitioners tested blood sugar levels from urine and called diabetes 'madhumeha', which means 'saccharine urine'.

Sour

Sour accentuates the taste of food. It is called amla in Sanskrit. It is derived from the earth and fire elements. It aggravates both pitta and kapha but soothes vata. Amla helps in the formation of saliva and subsequently forms digestive enzymes. It is light, hot and unctuous. It generates heat in the muscles and awakens the sensory organs of the body and faculties of the mind; it energizes and rejuvenates the body. When consumed excessively, it sensitizes the teeth, hardens the vocal cords and causes thirst. It can create pus in wounds, swelling, rashes and dryness in the skin.

Salty

Salty is lavana in Sanskrit. The word lavana also means graceful and tasteful. No matter how well cooked, spiced or seasoned food may be, it is tasteless without salt. Hence the meaning tasteful; it adds taste to the food. Lavana is hot and unctuous – it is made of fire and water elements. It fuels the digestive fire, soothes vata and liquefies kapha. Salt is an excellent cleanser – it softens the body tissues and has antibiotic properties. It removes fatigue, stiffness and swelling. When used inordinately, it aggravates pitta, robs the skin of its moisture (thereby causing early wrinkles), weakens the teeth and bones, causes prematurely grey hair and baldness, adversely affects sexual potency, dulls the senses and causes thirst, acidity and eczema. Yogic texts classify salt as rajas; therefore it contributes to restlessness of the mind and depression.

Pungent

Pungent is called katu in Sanskrit. It means acrid, stimulating and strongly scented as well. The taste of most peppers and chillies is pungent. It is chiefly derived from the fire and air elements. It promotes glandular, nasal and sweat secretions. It aids the digestive fire and stimulates the senses. Katu pacifies kapha and vitiates both vata and pitta. It has a detoxifying effect on the body. It produces antibodies, maintains the quality of blood, helps in the absorption of food, opens up the body pores (rejuvenating the skin) and adds taste to food. It is light, hot and rough. When consumed excessively, it weakens the glands, causes scrawniness, mental and sexual disorders and loss of thirst. In some cases, it can cause tremors and a burning sensation in the feet and hands.

Bitter

Tikta is bitter. Made from ether and air, bitter is an immuno-modulator, meaning it keeps your immune system in balance. It is excellent for the skin and blood. It is a natural cleanser and purifier. It absorbs moisture and burns body fat. It is an antidote, antitoxin, antihistamine and an enzymatic antigen. The ethereal and bitter properties of tikta aid digestion, and it acts as a blood purifier. It easily overpowers the other five tastes.

Tikta causes dryness in the mouth but often leaves a non-slimy taste. It pacifies pitta and kapha and vitiates vata. Too much tikta is detrimental to all the dhatus: it causes dryness in the skin, excessive thirst and fatigue. It kills appetite and causes incomplete bowel movement. If taken immoderately, it reduces the span of attention. Its immediate effect may make it appear to be a stimulant, but it almost always acts as a depressant. When it comes to taste, coffee fits the description of bitter almost perfectly.

Astringent

Made from the elements of earth and air, it is called kasaya in Sanskrit. It is healing; it promotes overall well-being and is calming. It sort of stiffens your mouth and throat, as if your mouth is shrivelled. It dries up your mouth and your tongue feels cold. It slows down the energy flow and checks gastritis. It reduces the production of urine and semen, and causes hard bowels. In people with any prior heart condition, it can also cause heartache. When taken excessively, it causes flatulence, mouth ulcers and spasms – even convulsions. In extreme cases, it can also cause hemiplegia (paralysis of one side of the body).

The six tastes have a natural tendency to move in a certain way. The tastes predominantly comprising air and fire tend to move up. For example, consumption of pungent and bitter tastes can cause reflux, mostly because air and fire are light and tend to move upwards. The tastes comprised of earth and water move downwards. They can slow down the metabolism and cause heaviness. The other tastes can move both ways. Any taste in excess always vitiates one, two or all three of the doshas. Tastes only support the body when enjoyed moderately. See the table below for the six tastes and their movements.

The Six Tastes and Their Movements

Taste	*Property*	*Elements*	*Movement*
Sweet	Heavy , unctuous, cold	Water, earth	Evenly spread
Sour	Hot, light, unctuous	Earth, fire	Downwards
Salty	Hot, unctuous	Fire, water	Downwards
Pungent	Light, hot, rough	Fire, air	Upwards
Bitter	Dry, rough	Air, ether	Upwards
Astringent	Dry, cold	Earth, air	Upwards

An important thing to know about the classification of the six tastes is that it strictly refers to the natural taste of a substance, and thus the individual classification of a food. If you mix a lot of sweet in a bit of sour and bitter, this may make the ultimate product sweet, but it won't act as sweet on your body.

For example, you can put honey in a cup of tea to make it sweet. But the tea can't be classified as sweet now, because this is not the natural sweetness of the tea. Therefore, you can't have tea and expect to gain the same results that come from consuming natural and wholesome honey.

Just as the colours red and yellow combine to make orange, and just as you cannot get the red and the yellow colours back from orange, two tastes mixed don't act individually on the body; their combination may have an entirely different effect than if the two were consumed separately.

Why do we crave certain foods over others? It's not just because of the taste. There are many foods that taste awful but still we consume them. What taste does beer or alcohol have? What about the sickly sweet maple syrup? Or the unique Vegemite? How a food tastes is only one aspect of its influence. What matters much more is how it acts on the body and the experience it triggers in our minds. It is this experience that makes us want to have certain foods more than others.

A food may be sour, and therefore hot and light, but its effect on the body may be sweet and soothing. In other words, the effect of a food on your body may be quite different from its taste. For example, if you drink a sugary beverage like cola, it may taste sweet, but its effect on the body is not sweet but astringent. It will not quench your thirst – it will make you even thirstier and may cause reflux.

THE FOUR STAGES OF FOOD

When a food is consumed, it goes through various stages during its processing, before its residue is expelled from the body. Imagine eating a chocolate-vanilla cake after a spicy meal. The cake will feel sweet while you are eating it. It will be gratifying. While in the stomach, it'll soothe at first. As your body starts to process it, its taste will change from sweet to sour. It will make you feel a bit thirsty and a bit restless. Post-digestion, it will have an influence on your physical and mental health. It may boost your sugar levels and make you feel hyper.

What is sweet in taste may not necessarily be sweet in action. What is acidic in nature may not work as such on the body. For example, lemons are sour in taste. Their taste has acidic properties, but their effect is alkaline on the body. To aid a better understanding of these properties, Ayurveda notes four stages of consumption. And at each stage, the food we consume has an impact on our physical and mental health.

Taste

Taste is the joy you get when food first touches your tongue. As you start to savour the various ingredients, they tickle your taste buds. There is a certain bliss. The sublime scent of basil, the piquancy of fresh mozzarella, the tanginess of the tomato sauce in your pasta, the aroma of freshly baked bread – they all enhance your sense of taste. When you bite into a juicy mango, or a sumptuous strawberry, or a sweetmeat like the gulab jamun, you are not eating food: you are experiencing it. Ayurveda uses the word rasa to indicate that taste, that joy. Rasa can evoke emotions, memories, feelings and reactions. It forms the primary basis of our food preferences.

No matter how nutritious a food may be, if you are not well disposed to its taste, you can't receive all of its benefits. In this context, taste is the predigestion stage; you are chewing the food and the saliva is infusing it with digestive enzymes. The food has not reached your stomach yet.

The chief effect at this stage is on your mental and emotional states. For example, most narcotics don't need to reach your stomach to achieve the desired result. Through their inhalation or aroma alone, they can trigger a whole range of thoughts and emotions within moments of their consumption. The taste, regardless of whether you snort it, lick it or suck it, is a significant factor. No matter how subtle its influence, rasa of a food is a vital factor. In the case of most intoxicants the effect is visible immediately, whereas with normal foods the effects build up over time.

It is for this reason that a healthy diet is supposed to have an agreeable taste. All sensory organs are capable of perceiving taste. It is not just the food itself that may taste delectable. An agreeable sound, a comforting touch, a delightful aroma and a delicious meal with an attractive form are also aspects of rasa, taste. These are the tastes for the various cognitive organs in your body.

The more that these tastes or sensory experiences are in harmony, the more positive is the effect of the food on you. That is why flavour, aroma, taste, presentation and ambience all make a difference to how your body accepts the food you eat.

For example, do a takeaway from your favourite restaurant. You'll notice eating that meal at home hasn't given you the same fulfilment as eating it in the restaurant. This is largely because at home you can't recreate the same experience or ambience. If it were just about the physical aspect of food, it wouldn't have mattered one bit where you ate it. But the truth is, where and how you eat your food has a bearing on the three subsequent stages of the food's influence on your body.

Potency

Once the food is past the taste buds, it ends up in the stomach. It leads to the second stage of the food's processing by the body. Whatever we can taste has a certain potency. It is called virya, also meaning strength or efficacy. Although this potency may be experienced by any of the five sensory organs, my present focus is on food being digested by the stomach. Potency of any food is realized during digestion. Virya specifically refers to the nature of food during the process of assimilation or digestion in the stomach.

It could be cold, hot, heavy, light, unctuous or rough. Broadly, it is classified as either hot or cold. Cold food will vitiate kapha and hot food will vitiate pitta. Whether it pacifies or deranges vata depends on your constitution and the time you consume such food. For example, milk is cold and heavy. It aggravates kapha and is heavy on digestion. If you take it in the morning, it does not vitiate vata, but if you drink milk after sunset it deranges vata and causes gas.

Virya refers to the essence of the substance. It is the influence of any food from the moment it reaches your stomach till the time the food is completely digested. In other words, it is the effect of a substance on your mind and body during the phase of digestion. For example, cabbage is cold and light in rasa but rough and hot in virya. It causes gas during the process of digestion no matter what time of the day it is consumed.

Maturity

If you notice carefully, after a food has been digested, some foods leave you feeling lethargic, whereas some make you feel energetic; some make you feel light and many make you feel heavy. This post-digestion effect is called the maturity of the food. After the food has been digested, but the residue has not been excreted, the food you have consumed is in the third stage called vipaka. It means ripening or maturing. It is the post-digestive state.

At this stage, both the food and its residue are in your system and are having an impact on your health. The residue in the stomach is producing toxins and the nutrients absorbed have not yet been fully transported throughout your body. Processed foods leave more residue in your body. Eating a cheese-and-tomato sandwich on white bread is not the same as eating a green salad with tomatoes, cheese and croutons in it. The latter will digest better, absorb better and leave you feeling better.

Foods that are sweet, salty or sour in vipaka are good at eliminating wind and help excretion of urine and stools. Foods with pungent, bitter and astringent vipaka aggravate vata and can cause irregular bowel movements and reproductive disorders.

All acidic foods, with the exception of citrus fruits, have pungent or bitter vipaka and should be avoided as much as possible. Naturally, citrus foods have sweet or sour vipaka and are really good for the body. Most dry fruits, for example, have hot vipaka and aggravate pitta.

Effect

This is the fourth and the final stage of the food's processing by the body. It is also known as the specific or net potency. The Sanskrit word is prabhava. Its literal meaning is effect. The food has been digested, the residue has been excreted, and the rest has been fully absorbed by your body. The food you consumed has shown its complete and net effect. Let's take the example of milk again – cow's milk in this case. Its taste is sweet and light, its potency is heavy and sweet, its maturity is unctuous and heavy, and its effect is acidic and light. So milk may help wash down spices after a meal, but its net effect is acidic and it vitiates vata.

Knowing all about food is not enough; we must know what, when and how to eat. I have known numerous patients who ate according to their constitution, who were strict vegetarians, who followed the rules of diet, yet were not in the best of health. Just like we can't transfer the contents of a full one litre bottle to another that is half its size, we can't absorb the living energy of our food if we don't align ourselves to that energy. I'm not referring to any esoteric aspects of food consumption. Instead, I wish to share with you simple and practical principles of eating our food, that will make all the difference between feeling healthy and feeling ill; between looking lustrous and looking listless.

The Eating Sense

Isha, a woman in her mid-thirties, was depressed. Her feelings were not unreasonable. She was overweight by twenty pounds and, despite all her efforts, couldn't lose weight. She'd tried all sorts of diet programmes. Every time she lost a few pounds, she gained them back quicker than she'd lost them. She'd tried fasting and supplements, she'd even become a vegetarian, but there was no improvement. Isha was happily married with no kids. The intriguing thing was that she was eating the right food in the right amounts, yet she was unable to lose weight. She asked me why God was so unkind to her.

'What's God got to do with your body weight?' I asked. She felt some negative forces in the universe were preventing her from permanently shedding weight. She told me that her dream was to be able to fit into certain dresses. She said she wanted to look beautiful in the mirror. I told her that she was beautiful but she wouldn't believe it. Her inability to lose weight had deeply affected her self-belief, self-confidence and self-esteem. She saw herself as a failure. She wasn't aiming to become a supermodel: all she wanted was to shed twenty pounds, she said. She asked me how it could be that no diet programme worked for her. She tried eating less, she tried eating more, she tried eating certain foods and she tried salad-only diets, but every time she lost weight, she put it back on.

She had been a non-vegetarian all her life, but in the past five years, she had even become a vegetarian, she said. She tried exercising but she could not find any method to permanently shed her excess weight. 'Please tell me the truth, Swami,' she said. 'Can you help me?'

'Yes,' I said. 'You see, Isha, exercising or diet programmes are never a permanent way of losing weight. Your weight has little to do with what or how much you are eating. And God can't help you in losing weight.'

'Then?'

'You need to know the art of eating. There's no problem with your selection of foods. Diet is not the problem, just the eating sense.'

I shared with her the long-forgotten eating sense: the art of choosing what, when, how and how much you put in your stomach. She seemed somewhat, but not fully, convinced. Nevertheless, she followed my method of eating food properly over the next three months and came back to report that she had lost twelve pounds. She said she felt happier and fitter because she was not torturing herself, and in spite of eating everything, she was still losing weight. Another four months later, she reported losing another ten pounds. She exceeded her target of losing twenty pounds. It's been more than a year and she hasn't regained any weight.

In this chapter, I'm sharing with you the fundamentals of eating or the 'eating sense' as I call it. It's the common sense way of eating your food. Regardless of your dietary preferences, even if you are a hard-core non-vegetarian, if you follow the principles I share with you here, you will feel fitter, healthier and happier.

Eating is not just about what you eat. What you eat matters, but how you eat matters a lot more. Eating your food is not an act but an art, a discipline, a science – even a framework with several elements – that influences how your body and mind process and absorb what you eat. Some people find it incredibly hard to make changes to their diet. Some so love their meat or fried foods, and for many others it is not possible to change their dietary habits because of social expectations or religious strictures. And that's okay. It's not the best scenario, but we can work with it.

Nothing is absolutely bad or absolutely good. Clearly, there are millions of healthy meat eaters. I have known many who even consumed alcohol and ate meat every day, yet lived well into their eighties. Much depends on your state of mind. If you are the worrying type or mostly stressed, even a cucumber can do you harm. You can't help being the worrying or the stressed type, you may say. And that's okay too as long as you follow the eating sense. It will help you feel lighter and healthier. You'll sleep better and you'll wake up fresh.

THREE TYPES OF EATERS

Think of eating as a ritual. You sit down, your food is on the table, you ready yourself to perform the ritual, you start eating and you finish a little while later. Not everyone eats their food in the same manner, however. Chewing your food well is one of the most important aspects of the eating sense.

When it comes to the ritual of eating, there are mostly three types of people: those who eat quickly and barely chew their food, those who eat at a moderate pace and chew their food well, and those who eat rather slowly. The eating styles of these three types may be described as follows.

The Dog

The animals who have always had to compete and contend for their food generally eat quickly. They are in a rush, because they are worried that someone may wrest their meal from them, interrupt them or stave them off.

The dog is a fast eater. If you observe a dog eating food, you'll realize that he's rarely eating in peace. He's constantly watching in ten directions while he's eating. He is worried; it is his natural disposition. Long before they were tamed, dogs, like packs of wolves, had to hunt their food and eat it before other powerful animals could steal it from them. They were not digesting their food, and the length of their intestine afforded them this luxury.

They are comfortable being restless and alert all the time. In fact, they are expected to be that way. They must wake up at the slightest noise. But human beings need rest and peace. We need some time off – mentally and physically.

This first type of eater is a fast eater and he is comparable to a dog. If you eat food in a rushed manner without chewing it, you are likely to have indigestion. Many people I meet are not even aware that they have indigestion. Reflux or acidity are not the only signs of indigestion. When your food sits in your abdomen for any more than three hours, you're suffering from indigestion. Ayurveda states that ninety-five per cent of ailments in the human body arise from the stomach. Not chewing your food well is the leading cause of all major ailments in the body including, but not limited to, diabetes, blood pressure and irregular bowel movements. You also may tend to overeat, which could lead to obesity as well.

If a person eats too fast, his stomach is always strained. The job that should have been done by the hard teeth is being done by the soft intestine. Your stomach is designed to bake and not grind; it's an oven, not a blender. The teeth are designed to bite and chew. When your stomach has to digest larger bits and chunks of food, undigested food remains in it for much longer. Your body has to secrete more enzymes to digest that food. It makes your internal environment highly acidic. It makes you lethargic, even fatigued. Undigested food creates toxins in your system; it is the primary cause of indigestion, migraine and heaviness. Sleep is supposed to freshen and rejuvenate you, but people who eat food quickly tend to wake up tired.

The Lion

Turn on the Discovery Channel and watch a pride of lions going for a kill and then eating it. Even when hunting, there's a certain grace in their motion; there are no haphazard movements. While eating, they eat as if they are savouring every bite. They are not stressed because, unlike other carnivores, no one can snatch a meal from them. They take their time while feasting on their game. Those who eat like lions are the finest eaters. They consume their food at a moderate pace and chew their food well.

The Cow

Countless times in the Himalayan villages, I had the opportunity to observe cows grazing. Numerous times

I saw the goats and sheep grazing too fast. Their tiny, beautiful mouths would pluck the grass in short and swift movements. But never once did I see a cow rushing to either graze or ruminate. They took their time – they took too much time, in fact. Taking too much time to eat is not good for us humans.

The digestive systems of those who eat very slowly have to work hard, like the cows, because most of their food is cold by the time it gets to their stomach. When food is below room temperature, your body has to heat up that food in order to break it down. It is important to note that eating slowly does not necessarily mean one is chewing one's food well. Many eat slowly because they are doing something else while they are eating: they may be reading, watching television, talking on the phone or working on the computer, etc.

You can only eat your food at the right speed if you are focussing on the food while you are eating. If you are doing any other activity while dining, it is not possible to maintain a healthy pace of eating and chew your food properly. Most people are not unhealthy because they are eating the wrong food. They are unwell because they are not eating it properly. Maintain a steady pace while eating – neither too fast nor too slow – and see your health improve by the day.

FIVE ASPECTS OF THE EATING SENSE

How you eat is an art. Each one of us practises it differently. You may have seen people who work stressful jobs and have challenges at home eat all sorts of stuff, yet maintain good health. If one is cheerful, carefree or contented, the role of diet loses much of its significance, because such people can digest practically anything. Due to their fine mental health, their bodies remain fit too. A good sense of eating has five aspects, namely mindfulness, water, quantity, gratitude and time. Let me elaborate.

Mindfulness

Most people overeat without realizing they are eating more than they should. The easiest way to know how much you should eat is to eat mindfully. Your body will tell you when it's had enough. To absorb the living energy of your food, mindfulness in your eating is essential. Mindfulness requires focussing on your food while you are eating it: savouring every bite, every morsel. Don't watch television, do any work or read while you are eating. In an ideal world, you shouldn't be holding any conversations, either. These are all distractions. Mindless eating leads to either eating too quickly or too slowly. If you eat mindfully and only eat when you are eating, you can almost never overeat, and you get the most from your food.

You can test this theory any day. Just go to your favourite restaurant on your own and order a meal. You will find yourself eating less than usual. This is because you are not holding a conversation while eating – you are simply focussing on your meal. Eating mindfully allows your mind to gain the most out of the food.

The second most important dimension of mindful eating is chewing your food well. Aim to be the lion – not in the selection of your food but in your manner of eating. Chewing well not only makes it easy on your stomach, it also helps you digest the food faster and actually makes the food more nutritious. When you chew food, the enzymes in saliva get mixed with the food. The more you chew, the more enzymes get mixed. When enzyme-rich, well-chewed food goes into your belly, your stomach processes it effortlessly. The food gets digested quickly and the body remains free of acids and toxins.

To those who can't give up their unhealthy diet, my only recommendation is to chew your food extremely well. Classical scriptures say that water should be *eaten* and food should be *drunk*. It means that whenever you are drinking water, you mustn't gulp it down. Take it sip by sip. And when eating, chew your food so well that it almost becomes liquid. The average human being has thirty-two teeth, so chew each bite a minimum of thirty-two times. Anyone chewing his food well is bound to be free of most physical ailments.

Water

More than 2300 years ago, India produced a brilliant mind: Chanakya. A superb economist and a philosopher, Chanakya also touched upon physical well-being in his works. He made a remarkable observation on water: 'When water is consumed half an hour before eating a meal, it is like holy nectar. When one drinks water during the meal, it works more like medicine. But drink it immediately after the meal, and it works as if poison.' The medical foresight in his statement is profound.

For centuries, modern science believed in drinking water immediately after a meal so that the food was washed down with a proper amount of water. This view is no longer valid, because research has long established that water ingested immediately after a meal leads to dilution of the gastric juices, causing indigestion. It creates an unnecessary burden on the liver and pancreas to secrete more enzymes.

When we drink water around twenty minutes before eating our food, it properly prepares the stomach. It activates the digestive enzymes, which better prepares the body to produce ample saliva and aids in more efficient and faster digestion. During the meal, it does no great harm, but gives no great benefit either. It is like medicine in the sense that it may act like a tonic by liquefying your meal in the stomach, thereby enabling better digestion. Immediately after food, though, it is harmful. It is like pouring icy water on a small campfire. If you drink water when your stomach is in the process of breaking down large chunks of your solid meal, it immediately dilutes the digestive enzymes. Your body has to work harder and longer to digest the food. And the colder the water, the greater the time it takes for food to digest.

Quantity

There can be no definitive one-size-fits-all guide on how much one should eat. Nevertheless, there are guidelines in Ayurveda. It states that you should eat in the one-third: one-third: one-third ratio. This means that one-third of your diet should be solid, one-third should be liquid and one third should be left in the stomach for air. The view in later texts was changed to half: one-fourth: one-fourth, meaning two parts of food, one part of water and one part of air.

It is important to leave one part for air so there is room to churn, mix, break down and digest the food. Think of a washing machine that is filled to the brim with clothes. The clothes won't wash well; you have to give them room to spin and churn. The same goes for your diet. Never eat to the full extent of your appetite. Always leave some room in your stomach.

According to modern science, hunger and satiety are based on the blood sugar levels. When the blood sugar level drops below a certain point, it creates the desire to consume food. When we consume food, gastric dilatation and increasing sugar levels tell us to stop. But when we eat unwholesome or processed foods, or when we eat quickly, by the time the brain realizes it is time to stop, we may already have eaten an excessive amount.

One of the remarkable qualities of wholesome foods (foods that are naturally nutritious), especially those rich in fat and protein, is that you cannot overeat them. You can over-drink sugary, fizzy, soft drinks but you cannot over-drink milk, for example. Your body knows how to break down natural foods, and it will tell you when it has had enough. If you practise mindful eating, you learn to listen to your body much better, and your body always tells you when to stop.

Gratitude

This may sound out of place, but never underestimate the importance of saying grace and expressing your gratitude before you start your meal. The Vedic view takes it even further. In the Vedas food is called God and God is food. The process of eating is considered a sacred ritual. It has been called yajna (sacred fire offerings). The digestive fire is the sacred fire burning in the pit of your stomach; each bite of food is an oblation and each sip of drink is a libation. This is in the temple of your body, at the altar of your soul. When you eat with this sentiment, food simply cannot harm you. From the most profound philosophical perspective, you befriend millions of micro-organisms in the food by eating like this; they enter your body to nurture you, nourish you and strengthen you.

In olden times in India, it was considered disrespectful and unhealthy to eat while sitting at the table. People would spread a thin mat and sit down on the floor. This was done out of gratitude: 'It is from the earth we have procured the food, so let's be in touch with the ground while partaking of its gifts.' They would set aside multiple bites of food for other beings in creation before eating the first one themselves. This was to thank the divine forces and to do their part of goodness.

Five grasas (mouthfuls) of offerings were set aside by every person – one each for the cow, the ancestors, a bird, a dog and another human being. Nature grows and thrives on the principle of sharing. Not only was grace said just before having food, often a meal was preceded by daily fire offerings or prayers. People would wake up, freshen up, bathe, offer water to the sun (I'll cover this bit later) and chant the Vedic mantras or say their daily prayers.

This instilled humility and calmness in them. It brought them in touch with the light within; it prepared their bodies and minds for food. Calm minds and bodies then extracted every vestige of nutrition and nourishment from the food they ate. Millions of people still follow this tradition in India. In the last decade or so, I don't remember any time I had food without offering it to the Divine first. It makes you feel complete.

Here's the simple practice: sit down at the table. Take a few deep breaths. Remind yourself that you work hard and do most things so you may enjoy a square meal. And, now that you have the meal in front of you, it's time to savour every bite. Thank God or nature or the universe for providing you with food. There are hundreds of millions of people on our planet who go to bed hungry every night. Remind yourself how lucky you are. Take a couple of sips of water. Pacify your body and your breathing. Just imagine you are doing fire offerings to the divine digestive fire in your stomach. Imagine that every morsel is a part of nature and that you are about to absorb this in you. Eat slowly, chewing every bite – enjoy the rasa in every morsel. This doesn't take more time; it simply takes awareness.

Time

Knowing when to eat is the greatest knowledge you can have when it comes to food. All Ayurvedic, yogic, tantric and other Vedic scriptures are in complete agreement regarding the best time to eat food. The morning mealtime may vary from person to person depending on their routine, but they strongly recommend having your dinner before sunset or just around that time. The consensus is to eat four hours before you go to sleep. Ideally, you should eat in the evening and then go for a walk. This is a simple recipe for a healthy life.

Eating just before going to bed is a definite way of aggravating the three doshas. Eating late or just before sleeping leads to weight gain. This is largely because your body secretes insulin when you eat just before sleeping, and insulin breaks down all nutrient groups – including proteins and carbohydrates – into triglycerides. Triglycerides are the primary type of fat found in the body and your diet.

Modern science validates this view by suggesting that the metabolism slows towards the end of the day. Even the secretion of insulin follows a pattern called the circadian rhythm. It decreases at night and is at the lowest point between midnight and 6 a.m., when it starts to rise again before hitting a peak between midday and 6 p.m.

With practice, it becomes easy to go to bed four or five hours after your meal, but if you can't fall asleep because you are hungry, you can have a light wholesome snack, like a fruit, an hour or so before going to bed. The goal is that you should go to bed with an empty stomach. If you do that, you sleep soundly, you wake up fresh, the doshas remain in balance, you don't feel thirsty in the middle of the night and your sleep is uninterrupted. It is particularly good for all kapha disorders.

Ayurvedic texts also state that one should only eat after the previous meal has been fully digested by the body. In other words, you should only eat when you feel hungry. If you eat the right quantity and chew it well, you'll feel like eating something every three hours. Have a light wholesome snack. If you take water at regular intervals, your body will send you the hunger signal at just the right time. It is not prudent to stay hungry for long periods, because your body starts to use your natural energy reserves, and then when food hits your abdomen, the excess release of energy is converted into fat.

Irregular mealtimes are a great contributor to obesity. It is equally damaging for your health to keep stuffing yourself when you already have food in your stomach. Yogic texts state that any good food digests completely within four hours at the most, no matter how sedentary your lifestyle is. If you don't feel hungry four hours after your previous meal, the chances are that the food is not digested yet. And when your food is not digested four hours after it has been eaten, it is most definitely producing toxins in your body.

SEASONS AND DIET

Your body undergoes an inner transformation when the seasons are changing. Your immune system is weak at these times. It takes time for the body to adjust. This is why during spring and just before the onset of winter, seasonal allergies are at their worst. If you enter a season healthy, you are more likely to remain healthy throughout the season. And this isn't just true for physical health – it is also true for mental health. If you start a season in a depressed mood, you are likely to spend the next three months in melancholy.

There are two stints of nine nights, called Navaratra, that come twice a year at the time of the cusp of seasons. Navaratras are widely celebrated in India. These nine nights are considered the festive nights of Mother Divine. Mother Nature is Mother Divine. During this period, people stay mostly indoors and avoid eating any food that is cooked outside in restaurants. They go on a gluten-free diet consisting of only cow's milk, fruits and certain vegetables. Some also fast completely for the whole nine days, subsisting on just a liquid diet of fruit juices.

It has been observed that these people may completely avoid seasonal allergies. Every time there is a change in season, there is a festival in India. The seasons are not four but six in Vedic scriptures, namely spring (vasanta), summer (grishma), rainy (varsha), autumn (sharada), winter (hemanta) and the cool season (shishira). The purpose of the festivals is to express gratitude to Mother

Nature and introduce the new foods of the season in a cheerful manner. How a food is introduced can be the decisive factor in whether your body accepts or rejects it. For example, if you force a child to eat a certain food, and he doesn't like it, he may develop a lifelong repulsion towards that food.

Vata ailments (meaning all disorders arising out of vata) – especially seasonal allergies – germinate in the body during the summer; they get vitiated in the rainy season and pacified in autumn.

Pitta afflictions accumulate during the spring; they are aggravated in the summer and pacified in autumn.

Kapha accumulates in the body from the dawn of winter but doesn't manifest its disorders till the spring. It is pacified in the summer. See the table below for the relationship between doshas and the seasons.

Doshas and Seasons

	Accumulates	Aggravates	Pacifies
Vata	Summer	Rainy	Autumn
Pitta	Spring	Summer	Autumn
Kapha	Winter	Spring	Summer

Your constitutional disorders are likely to be in the seasons as per the humours above. It is best to go on a light diet during the change of seasons. Light means avoiding all processed, fried, fatty and fast foods. Ideally, you should be on a gluten-and-dairy-free diet for one week during a change of season. This is the easiest way to avoid many seasonal allergies and physical weaknesses.

The food you eat may have any of the six tastes; it may be hot or cold, oily or dry, hard or soft, liquid or solid or semi-solid. It may be chewable, lickable, drinkable, suckable; it may be nutritious or junk. There are numerous other properties of food. Ultimately, however, the real nature of the food you consume can be ascertained by considering its two crucial aspects: light or heavy and acidic or alkaline. Either it is heavy to digest or it is light to digest. And the food acts either as acidic or as alkaline on your body. If you consume foods that are light on your digestion and alkaline in nature, you naturally remain healthier.

What to Eat

For years I researched the issue of nutrition. I tried to align the Ayurvedic dietary guidelines and the modern system of nutrition. I worked with my doctors to understand the implications of various foods for various people; I experimented with foods based on the constitution of an individual. What I found was nothing short of startling. While Ayurveda is extremely accurate in determining which foods vitiate various doshas, it is not the physical nature of the food but its tendency (svabhava) that has the most impact on patients.

There were some kapha patients who didn't respond well to yogurt, and there were just as many who did, for instance. This was intriguing. But there was no confusion once we considered the alkaline or acidic nature of various foods and the natural tendencies of such foods. Now we could arrive at a simple food chart that could be used by anyone.

Appendix 1 of the book presents two lists of acidic and alkaline foods, with the categorization of goodness (sattvic), passion (rajasic) or ignorance (tamasic). The more alkaline and sattvic foods you consume, the healthier you become. Additionally, if you take care of the quantity, time and manner of eating, you are most unlikely to fall sick. This is one way of ensuring good health: eat wholesome foods at the right time, in moderate quantities and with a sense of gratitude.

Ayurveda recommends a balanced diet – a sattvic diet. In line with the modern system of nutrition, it suggests that our food should be healthy. But it also places an emphasis on the food being sattvic, and also on its tastefulness and its agreeableness with one's body. There are five important terms in Ayurveda, namely, fat (sneha), protein (snigdha), tasty (rasya), agreeable (hridya) and carbohydrates (madhura, literally sweet).

Although the terms sneha and snigdha literally mean oil and gluten, in terms of their effect on the body (the fourth stage of food), they are identical to fats and proteins. Five thousand years ago, most people were routinely engaged in physical labour. Therefore, Ayurveda recommended that a diet should have a decent proportion of carbohydrates, because the human body directly derives energy from carbohydrates to sustain work. And the rishis reasoned that anything with sweetness in it will contain carbohydrates. The sweeter the food, the more the carbohydrates. Even bread, rice and milk have a natural sweetness, because they all have carbohydrates.

The rishis didn't stop at nutrients alone. They stated that for us to receive the optimum benefit from food, it must be tasty. If we dislike the food we have to eat, we put ourselves under stress. And when we are stressed, our brains release a whole heap of chemicals that have an adverse effect on our digestion. These chemicals withdraw the proteins from the gastrointestinal tract and direct them to the hypothalamus – a region of the brain that regulates body temperature, thirst, hunger and other homeostatic systems – thus leading to indigestion. All of this can be avoided if food is tasty.

Further, as I've explained earlier, some foods sit well with us while others don't. Some of us can digest milk easily, whereas some others are highly lactose intolerant, for example. This is called hridya – agreeableness of the food in Ayurveda.

To find the right foods, start by listening to your body. Your body has an infallible feedback system. It tells you what is sitting well with it and what's not. As long as your diet is balanced, you will continue to feel energetic and healthy. I frequently meet people who are well into their eighties but extremely fit. They are mostly vegetarians and have eaten a basic but healthy diet throughout their lives. They have no Parkinson's disease, no Alzhiemer's disease, no diabetes, no hypertension and no heart disease. In fact, they are not on any medication. They journey from distant places to my ashram; they do a trek of forty minutes and cross a river. If you look at them, you will guess their ages to be in the mid-sixties.

These are not people who have consulted Ayurveda for their dietary needs. They haven't even taken vitamin supplements. They have just lived a life of physical and mental purity. There is one more factor in common. They have all eaten a diet of sattvic foods that are alkaline. This is the basis of their health and longevity. Let me elaborate on acidic and alkaline foods.

ACIDIC AND ALKALINE FOODS

In Ayurveda, acidic foods are called amla and alkaline foods are called kshara. Understanding the pH factor is paramount for determining which foods are acidic and which are alkaline. The earliest pH testing methods involved burning a substance at a high temperature and reading the residue to ascertain the pH. Five thousand years ago, while they did not have the sophisticated testing methods and tools available to modern science, they were remarkably insightful.

Ayurveda was surprisingly advanced. It understood that while burning a substance to test for its acidity was a viable method of testing, this was only one way of doing so. Ayurvedic practitioners would caramelize some substances, squeeze others, extract some and press many to understand the nature of the essence of that food. In its truest sense, this is what alchemy is: understanding the essence of matter to utilize it for consumption, transmutation or treatment purposes. The amount of butter and cream you can get from milk, for instance, can accurately determine its fat content. If you heat milk and 'split' it, it turns into a type of curd cheese like ricotta called paneer (the Indian cheese). This allows you to gauge the protein content of the milk.

The sage-physicians of Ayurveda didn't call acidity and alkalinity pH, they called it vipaka (the effect of the food – the fourth stage of the food). They figured that madhura or kshara vipaka (alkaline effect) bestowed the finest health on a person. Therefore, Ayurveda greatly emphasized the consumption of alkaline foods. Most alkaline foods are highly sattvic in nature; they promote mental and physical well-being.

All meats, intoxicants, condiments, processed and canned foods are very acidic. Modern science considers dairy mostly acidic, but Ayurveda considers all dairy products generated from cow's milk to be alkaline. All herbs, spices and most vegetables are alkaline. Avocados and coconuts are very alkaline, as are rock salt, sprouted beans and vegetables like spinach, cucumber and broccoli. Kemp (sea vegetable), horseradish and miso are very alkaline. All citrus fruits are acidic before ingestion but they act alkaline on the body during and after ingestion.

In this day and age, we are obsessed with data, but the truth is that selection of foods is a natural, simple and instinctive process. Your mind and body will tell you if a certain food is good for you or not. An acidic diet aggravates vata and pitta. Alkaline foods pacify all the three doshas. Indian gooseberry (amlaki or amla as it is commonly known) is a very alkaline food. It pacifies vata, pitta and kapha. It is sour but leaves a sweet, honey-like aftertaste in the mouth. All alkaline foods are light in digestion and their effect is soothing or cooling (sheetala) on the body.

The pH Factor

From the current scientific perspective, the pH value is the sole factor in determining whether a food is acidic or alkaline and how acidic or alkaline it is. The modern concept of pH has been around for more than a century, in fact. A Danish chemist, Søren Peder Lauritz Sørensen, invented the pH scale in 1909. pH values exist at the fluidal, glandular and cellular levels and in the tissues and organs. Each individual cell in your body has a pH level. pH stands for potential for hydrogen. It refers to the concentration of hydrogen ions. The fewer the hydrogen ions, the greater the pH level; the greater the pH level, the more the alkalinity. Your cells, tissues or fluids could be acidic, alkaline or neutral.

Measured on a scale of 0–14, anything above 7 is alkaline and anything below 7 is acidic. A pH reading of 7 is neutral. When the three doshas are in balance, your body is in a state of homeostasis. You achieve this outcome by maintaining the acid–alkali balance in your body. In other words, maintaining a pH between 7 and 8 is ideal for your body.

Every food you consume has an acid–alkali status. Acids generate hydrogen ions and alkalis absorb them. The greater the concentration of hydrogen ions in a substance, the more acidic it is. A higher pH means more alkaline. This is what you need in your diet – higher pH. Hydrogen ions are positively charged particles. They are highly unstable, active and reactive. They attach to a protein and are capable of completely modifying its structure.

People with low pH levels age quickly, because skin, hair and most muscles are made from protein. pH is measured in molecular weight also known as moles per litre. An increase of one point on the pH scale represents a tenfold or one thousand per cent decrease in the concentration of hydrogen ions. And a decrease of one point on the pH scale means a thousand per cent increase in hydrogen ions. Therefore, the difference between a pH of six and eight is not merely two points but a twentyfold change.

The Natural Mechanism

Over millions of years, the human body has evolved to be an extraordinarily intelligent system. There are three primary organs that maintain the acid–alkali balance in your body. They are your lungs, kidney and skin. In addition, your body has a buffer system made up of proteins or phosphate-containing molecules that try to maintain a pH balance in various bodily fluids.

The process of metabolism produces a number of gaseous acids. Most notably, carbon dioxide mixes with water to produce carbonic acid. The process of respiration flushes out these acids. Yogic texts place great emphasis on regulation of breath. Deep breathing is the easiest way to flush out the gaseous toxins. Shallow breathing is synonymous with ill health, according to Ayurvedic texts. Contemporary medical science supports this view, as shallow breathing leads to a condition called respiratory acidosis. It causes hypoventilation (abnormally decreased speed and depth of breathing) and retention of carbon dioxide, directly harming one's health.

In olden times, householders started their day by offering oblations to the sun while standing in a river or a pond. This reduced the positively charged particles in their bodies, thereby keeping acidity in check. Your body produces a lot of acids while you are sleeping, especially if you eat just before bedtime. After the oblations, they would breathe deeply twenty times. This produced an instant alkaline effect on the volatile or gaseous acids in the body. The yogis were required to do meditation and deep breathing before even leaving their beds. This is the first thing true yogis do even today.

All the acids in the bloodstream produced by metabolism are filtered by the kidneys. While the lungs filter the gaseous acids, kidneys filter the fixed acids, notably uric acid. Shaped like a bean, your kidneys are not much bigger than your thumb. The kidney tissues are quite tender. If your acid intake is too high for the kidneys to tackle on their own, they borrow reserve base compounds from the bones and muscles. Strong body odour is usually a clear sign that you are on an acidic diet. Over a period of time, an acidic diet will rob your muscles of their suppleness and may cause osteoporosis. If it doesn't lead to osteoporosis, it will certainly weaken your bones. It is worth noting that the pH of most alcoholic drinks ranges between 3 and just over 5. They can play havoc with your kidneys.

What lungs do with respiration, your skin does with perspiration; it flushes out the acids. The amount is not significant, nevertheless anything is better than keeping those acids inside your body. In Ayurveda, the benefits of abhyangama (massage) have been stated in abundance. Massage is also another way of making your skin more responsive, strong and healthy. It gives life and lustre to your skin. The healthier your skin, the better its capability to breathe. Perspiration of skin is its respiration.

Alkaline diets lead to healthier skin; you remain young longer. Premature wrinkles, lines, freckles and dryness are the signs of an acidic body. Ayurveda states that your skin has seven layers. Cosmetics, no matter how good they are, can only take care of the first three layers – at most. If you really want healthy skin, that is breathing and strong at all seven layers, an alkaline diet is your best bet. It is extremely difficult to avoid wrinkles with a highly acidic diet.

While acid–alkali imbalance is at the root of almost all physical diseases, excess acidity or alkalinity can lead to either of two conditions in the body.

Acidosis

As it is, the human body is acidic in nature. All secretions are basically acidic. Most secretions in the body have an element of heat; they are designed to either break down, digest or absorb various substances. Even saliva is acidic in nature. From rasa to shukra (saliva to semen), they are all acidic in nature. The essence of semen – sperm – is alkaline, though. Prostatic secretion is acidic while seminal vesicular fluid (which comprises the greatest proportion of semen) is alkaline. Stress and diet can make it vary, though. All glandular secretions are acidic in nature and the human body is constantly producing them. Therefore, it is all the more important to soothe your body through alkaline foods.

When you deprive your body of the minimum alkaline needs and your body continues to produce metabolic acids, it leads to a build-up of these acids in your body. This condition is known as chronic low-grade metabolic acidosis. Acidosis hardens your arteries, weakens your bones and kidneys, spoils your skin and affects your well-being. Think of the ring in the bathtub. After you have bathed, the acid in the water leaves marks on the bathtub. Similarly, if you consume an acid-rich diet, the acidic residue remains in your system, and it is a burdensome job for your kidneys to cleanse it. Not to mention the additional load on your digestive system. This acidic residue is called ama (pronounced aama) in Ayurveda (explained in more detail later in this book).

With age, as the kidneys become weaker, acidosis gets worse. Metabolic acidosis can also be caused by insufficient production of bicarbonate. Bicarbonate is a natural alkaline chemical produced by your body. Renal (kidney) problems, and gastrointestinal conditions like diarrhoea and pancreatic disorders, can also cause the loss of bicarbonate. Dietary negligence or ignorance, however, is the foremost cause of metabolic acidosis. Therefore, the easiest way to fix acidosis is by changing your diet.

Cola drinks, for example, have a pH level of around 2.5. This is extremely acidic. To neutralize one glass of cola in your body, you would need to drink thirty glasses of water. Acidosis can lead to chronic headaches, sleepiness or even insomnia, vertigo, seizures, diarrhoea, shortness of breath, chronic cough, palpitation, indigestion, reflux, heartburn, loss of calcium in the body, weakness in the bones, dry skin and other skin disorders including rashes, acne, body odour, increased risk of formation of kidney and bladder stones, accelerated ageing, degenerative diseases, fatigue and hormonal and glandular disorders. And I have only just scraped the surface here.

When your cellular pH level goes outside the normal range (7.3–7.5), your enzymes work a hundred per cent harder to restore the balance. Enzymes are the basis of all metabolic functions in the body. An acid–alkali imbalance leads to enzymatic malfunction. It prepares the perfect breeding ground for chronic physical and mental disorders. While I am at it, let me state that antacids may relieve the symptoms of heartburn in the short term, but they are extremely damaging in the longer term. They confuse and weaken your digestive system and promote acidity in the body.

It's much better to regulate your diet to avoid heartburn than to consume antacids. They are not really antacids; they are pro-acids, because in the longer term they create an acidic environment in your stomach and wreak havoc on your intestine. Their relief is entirely symptomatic and therefore temporary. When you repeatedly use medicines to suppress the secretion of stomach acids, it can create a highly toxic, even cancerous, environment in the stomach. One of the easiest things to do to avoid heartburn – which is merely a symptom of acidosis – is to go to bed on an empty stomach.

Alkalosis

As you may have guessed, alkalosis is the opposite of acidosis. It can also pose health risks. It is a rare condition, and I am only mentioning it here to give you a complete picture. It is almost impossible to have alkalosis by eating a balanced, common-sense diet. In other words, you need not worry about alkalosis if you are consuming food with a high pH level. Your body is producing enough acids, so a moderate amount of alkali-rich food cannot do you any harm.

People suffering from alkalosis are generally the ones who take certain drugs to maintain their body's alkaline state. High dosages or prolonged use of such drugs can cause alkalosis. As I mentioned earlier, antacids promote alkalinity in the body, but it is a terrible method of doing so. They completely disrupt the body's natural homeostasis, by achieving temporary and artificial increase in pH levels. The damage caused by them is permanent and organic.

Certain gastrointestinal disorders can also cause alkalosis, but this is fairly unusual. The yogis of olden times always preferred to stay in the mountains, in the high altitudes, because the low levels of oxygen and the low temperatures there slow down the metabolic processes and secretions, creating a healthy and alkaline environment for the body. The yogis could remain physically fit in these regions by eating frugally.

There are various ways to test your body's pH levels, but to be frank, testing your pH level is a little obsessive, in my view. You should simply eat a balanced diet. The definition of balance is that your diet should consist of eighty per cent alkaline foods and twenty per cent acidic foods. In the ideal world, one hundred per cent of your diet should be alkaline, because your body is already producing enough acids. For most people, though, it is not possible to go on a completely alkaline diet, for a variety of reasons. So, you should at least go for the eighty-twenty rule.

By following this dietary philosophy – and other principles and practices outlined in this book – your chances of remaining healthy increase exponentially. Is it possible to completely avoid disease in our bodies, though? Or, more importantly, what actually causes disease? If I eat the proper foods according to my constitution, if I maintain an alkaline diet, does it guarantee that I'll remain free of diseases? The answer is no. There's more to diseases than the food we ingest. There's no doubt that your chances of falling sick are almost negligible if you follow the eating sense, yet there's still a chance. For that, we must have a holistic understanding of what causes diseases beyond food and how we can avoid them. When I say 'I'm sick', who is actually sick in me?

10

Life Cycle of a Disease

'Disease then is a force and not matter.'
— Sushruta.

What is a disease, really? In the Oxford Dictionary of English, 'disease' is defined as: 'a disorder of structure or function in a human, animal, or plant, especially one that produces specific symptoms or that affects a specific location and is not simply a direct result of physical injury'.

Complete as that definition sounds, it is not how Ayurvedic or yogic scriptures look at it. A disease is not merely a structural or a functional disorder; it could easily be an emotional one also. Beyond the symptom-driven definitions in contemporary medical science, a disease is what disrupts your equilibrium, that is, your physical, mental, emotional and spiritual balance.

Self-deprecation is a disease, as is pride; anger is a disease, as is envy. Anything that throws you off-balance, physically or mentally, is a disease. It is when both body and mind are in balance — with each other and within themselves – that we can truly say one is healthy, that one is disease-free.

The great physician-sage, Sushruta, is asked in *Sushruta Samhita*, a major Ayurvedic text: 'What is a disease? What is it in a human that actually falls sick? What do we actually treat with medicines? Is it the body or the mind?'

Sushruta speaks: 'Anything that afflicts the inner man is disease; and that disease has its primary seat in the inner spring of vitality from which it flows out to the surface, the external body.'

The inner man is called the self or purusha in yogic texts. Pura means city. This body is a city of nine gates (the nine orifices) and the one that has the stronghold of this body is called purusha. When this purusha leaves the body, the person is pronounced dead. The atoms are there, the molecules are there, but there is no breathing, no movement, no emotions or feelings and no consciousness. Biologically, the body is intact, but it has lost the ability to maintain its individual nature within nature. It must now decompose and give back the five elements to nature. Even mentally or emotionally, when we lose our sense of individuality, we become listless, and life seems pointless. It is to retain this individuality that the powerful want more power, and the rich want more riches. The sense of individuality that comes from writing a fine poem, or winning a chess game, or finishing a painting, or beating a record, is the primary driving force behind the evolution and growth of our race.

The vital life force that gives us individuality – that gives us the ability to sustain ourselves as a separate entity while being a part of nature – is called the inner being or purusha. This is our centre of vitality, the control centre.

Sushruta Samhita further states that diseases spring from the afflictions of the inner man and then out to the body. I quote:[*]

> In man, as in everything else in the universe, the direction of the inherent force is from the centre to the circumference. The shock is felt first at the centre of vitality, whence it is transmitted outwards and thus affects the energy which holds the molecules together, dvyanuka and tryanuka (binary and tertiary atoms) of which the physical body is composed, and further opposes the dissolution of those molecules into their elemental constituents in the living organism.
>
> Even in cases of external injuries such as snakebite etc., the potency of the virus is carried at once to that centre from whence it is almost instantaneously transmitted through the external channels of the body to its surface, otherwise what purpose does the vayu (vital energy or nerve force) serve in the human economy? What do those myriads of chaitanya-vahini nadis (sensory nerves, literally, nerves carrying consciousness) exist for in the human system?
>
> In all diseases the subjective sensations are the first to be experienced. 'I am ill', 'I feel hot', etc., are the voices of sensations, which form the basis of the disease. Disease then is a force and not matter.

The passage above contains two incredible insights. First, anything that afflicts the inner being is a disease. The inner being is the one that experiences pain and pleasure, joy and sorrow; the one that is the essence of your life. The

---

[*] Translated by Kaviraj Dvarakanath Sen, edited and published by Kaviraj Kunja Lal Bhishagratna, printed by J.N. Bose, College Square, Calcutta, 1907.

state of your physical health and the state of your mental health both affect the inner being. Second, disease is a force and not matter. Both diseases and afflictions arise out of resistance. The body of a person who suffers from hay fever, for example, produces mucus. It does so because it believes that pollens are foreign material and must not be allowed inside the body. A body that has no seasonal allergy accepts the foreign material and there is no resistance.

Disease is a resistance of the opposing forces in your body. The result of this resistance could be anything from formation of mucus or pus, to more serious cysts or lumps and ulcers, to terminal illnesses; cancers, strokes, haemorrhages and heart attacks. Although you are born with a certain constitution – and this is a powerful factor in determining your degree of resistance – the truth is that your health is chiefly in your own hands. You can elevate your physical and mental state so that you become resistance-free. When there is no resistance with the forces of nature, when there is no inner conflict of emotions and thoughts, you become healthy naturally.

FIVE CAUSES OF A DISEASE

According to Ayurveda, all diseases in the human body are due to one or more of the five causes listed below.

Unwholesome Thoughts and Actions

There is a term in Ayurveda called prajna-aparadha. Prajna means wisdom or intellect and aparadha means fault or transgression. On par with poor diet in its detriment to good health, this is considered the original cause of disease in a human being. Impure thoughts and unwholesome actions originating from such thoughts are called prajna-aparadha; they vitiate all three doshas. Overindulgence or suppression of natural urges, immoral and unrighteous conduct, lack of modesty and compassion, friendship with the wicked, jealousy, hatred, anger, fear, greed and lack of discipline and enthusiasm are deemed intellectual errors. Excessive, negative and perverted use of your body, speech and mind are prajna-aparadha according to Ayurveda. These almost invariably lead to physical and mental disorders.

Unwholesome Diet

Ayurveda lists seven aspects of an unwholesome diet. They are prakriti (your constitution), svabhava (nature of the food), karana (how it's prepared), samyoga (combination of various ingredients), rasi (amount of food being consumed), desa (place where it's being consumed) and kala (time of consumption).

Errors and imbalances in these seven aspects are the leading cause of disease. They also adversely affect a person's mental state. If you have read, understood and absorbed the earlier elucidation on your body, food and eating in this book, you know exactly what an unwholesome diet is. In a nutshell – foods that are against your own constitution, acidic and tamasic foods, irregular eating, immoderate consumption, processed, canned and fried foods, and overeating and late eating make for an unwholesome diet.

Time

During the changing seasons, your body is at its weakest. Vata gets vitiated in the rainy season, pitta is vitiated in summer and kapha is vitiated in spring, for instance. Based on your own constitution, it is particularly important to pay attention to your diet at the cusp of seasons. It is one of the greatest preventative measures you can take to stay healthy. The time factor in Ayurveda also refers to the time when you eat. Eating before sunset or four hours before you go to sleep is highly recommended. Eating late also vitiates kapha and vata. Ideally, you should go to bed on an empty stomach.

Ageing

The body naturally becomes weaker as one ages. The kidneys, heart, intestine, muscles, bones all weaken. The skin loosens and wrinkles, and the sympathetic and parasympathetic nervous systems become weaker. Memory loss, hair loss and loss of appetite are normal. As is infirmity – physical and mental. With ageing, doshas accumulate and vitiate much more quickly. It becomes harder to pacify them with medicine. It is in these later years that you will harvest the rewards of the care you took of your body in your youth.

If you eat and live healthily when you are young, you have much less to worry about with ageing. I have known people who smoked and played soccer, and said that their bodies were strong enough to endure the ill effects of smoking; that smoking did them no harm. This was until the day they could not even walk quickly, let alone run on the soccer field, while their non-smoking peers played three times a week. Your body can take a lot of ill-treatment when you are young. From unhealthy diets to impure thoughts, it can handle almost anything. But it all adds up and brews at the core of the consciousness, waiting to burst like a volcano when your body or mind grows weaker with age.

While ageing cannot be avoided, you can certainly delay it with wholesome living: a right mindset and a right diet. A noble mind helps you to age gracefully. This is the best you can do with ageing – make it graceful.

Fate

Ayurveda lists fate as one of the factors that can as easily be the cause of a disease as any of the other four factors. The term used is daivam. It means your fate that is linked to your karmic cycle. Just like the fruit on trees, karma matures in its own time. Matured karma is called prarabdha. Like ripe fruit, it must fall from the tree.

It is through fate that Ayurveda explains why an infant, who has no karma in this lifetime – who is born to perfectly fit parents with great genetics – may still be born disabled or ill. The other four factors have not played a part yet in this child's life, so Ayurveda, intricately linked to Vedic thought, places such mysteries in the bucket of fate.

I am reminded of a real-life incident. Not too long ago, there was a healthy young man living in a small town in India. He was driving his motorcycle and wearing a helmet that only covered his head like a hat. He yawned while riding, and at that very moment a wasp flew straight into his open mouth. Enraged and agitated, it stung his tongue, just below the uvula. The man stopped the motorcycle, but within moments, his tongue swelled and blocked the passage of air; he choked and died on the spot before anyone could do anything about it. Such an incident can only be ascribed to fate.

Ayurveda recognizes that no matter how perfect a physician, patient or the treatment may be, it is nature alone that heals. Therefore, Ayurvedic texts specifically list fate as one of the five factors for causing disease. This may hurt our egos: we don't want to believe that there are certain aspects of our lives, of our physical bodies, that we have no control over. But upon deeper reflection, we can only conclude that listing fate as the fifth cause of disease is inherently reasonable.

The Four Killers

Diseases do not appear in the body overnight and consequently can't be cured in a jiffy. There is always a cause, a point of origin. Charaka wrote that the consumption of unwholesome foods is the primary cause of disease in the human body. This also includes negative emotions, which are unwholesome food for the mind. Our body is the primary seat of consciousness. Imagine standing in a beautifully decorated room that has a box in a corner full of putrefying meat. The smell of the rotting flesh will overpower your senses, and it'll become increasingly hard to even breathe in the room, much less sit in it and appreciate its beauty.

Similarly, the body becomes unfit when the consciousness is stinking. Unfitness of the body could occur in the form of its malfunctioning, diseases, a lack of strength or other physical disorders. When you are unable to let go of negative emotions, the consciousness starts to reek after a while. Ayurveda maintains that disease is the disequilibrium of dhatus.

Just like a termite can devour the healthiest wood, there are four aspects of our physical and mental disequilibrium that destroy our health. These are the four killers. They don't kill us overnight. They take their time, but they certainly rob us of our physical and mental health. With a bit of discipline, some understanding, mindfulness and dietary regulation, they can be removed from our system. Let me elucidate the four killers.

AMA

Here is the basic Ayurvedic principle: the food you cannot digest will eventually start to digest you. The digestive fire that hasn't received the right food to break down will start to break you down. Like a parasite, ama slowly eats away your health and eventually is the seed of all chronic problems. A knowledge of Ayurveda would be incomplete without understanding the concept of ama.

As mentioned earlier, acidic foods are called amla in Ayurveda. It is derived from the word ama. Ama means many things, but above all, it means toxic residue. No matter what you eat, it gets broken down into the core nutrients. There are only five things your body can absorb, namely, fat, protein, carbohydrates, vitamins and minerals. Anything that does not undergo complete transformation is residue. Any residue in the body is ultimately toxic; its very nature is acidic. Ama is produced either on account of indigestion or the excessive intake of acidic foods. It is a viscid and sludgy material with a pale yellow hue. The white deposit on your tongue is ama. One look at your tongue, and you can immediately know the state of your ama and your body's acid–alkali balance. The more toxic your body, the thicker the formation of ama on your tongue.

Heavy, rough, cold and overcooked foods create ama.

All tamasic foods are highly ama creating, and all rajasic foods are moderately ama creating. Most sattvic foods create practically no ama. In other words, acidic foods create ama and alkaline foods remove it from your system. Ayurveda states that negative emotions create ama as much as food does. It means that you may be eating a wholesome meal, but if you are mentally indisposed, your body will continue to house toxic residues. Of the many emotions, Ayurveda specifically notes passion, anger, greed, envy, grief, vanity and fear as ama-creating mental states.

Ama is the white matter on your tongue; it's the plaque on your teeth; it's the fat that clogs your arteries. It causes heartburn, gastritis and reflux. Obesity is the result of ama, as is cancer. It can exist at the cellular level, in the tissues, the glands or the organs. Cellular ama could result in anything from simple skin problems to the more grave cancer. In pitta people, it can lead to body odour, indigestion, stomach ulcers, gastritis and almost all the other gastrointestinal disorders. In kapha people, it can cause bronchitis, diabetes and heart disease. In vata peope, it can cause migraine, severe headaches, respiratory problems, bad breath and fatigue.

The presence of ama leads to stupor, weakness, lethargy, loss of appetite, fever and pain in the body, irritability, lacklustre skin, dark rings around the eyes, unclear urine, mucus in the stools, hard stools, constipation, coughing, lack of taste for food, poor digestion, insomnia, sleep apnoea and difficulty in waking from sleep. People with higher levels of ama are more prone to allergies, and they tend to catch a cold several times a year.

The easiest way to reduce ama is to follow the principles outlined in the chapter titled 'The Eating Sense' (Chapter 8). In a nutshell, if you are eating alkaline foods that are mostly sattvic, and you are eating with discipline and in moderation, ama will no longer be your worry. Other methods to eliminate ama include physical cleansing (covered later in this book in Chapter 13).

INDIGESTION

The second most potent killer is indigestion. Imagine a tree laden with fruits, its boughs extend several feet; its leaves are a lush green; its trunk is solid and wide – all in all, it is a healthy tree. Then, a strange affliction grips the tree; its fruit is infested with worms and its leaves are riddled with holes. You cannot possibly treat every single leaf and fruit – you have to get to the root cause of what is affecting the tree. Treating leaves and fruits is exactly what modern allopathic medicine does. And this is where you ought to know Ayurveda's view: ninety-five per cent of diseases have their roots in the digestive system. If you have good digestion, even ama is taken care of.

The only real disease in the physical body is poor digestion. A sensitive stomach is the primary cause of other physical ailments in the body. This is where the greatest toxins are produced. If your digestion is fine, you can almost be certain to live a long and a healthy life. If your digestion is in order, you can't be obese; you can't have stomach ulcers, asthma, heartburn, sleep apnoea and other sleeping disorders, headaches, migraine, pains in the joints, clogged arteries, mental and physical fatigue, phlegm, constipation, hard or irregular bowel movements and many other afflictions. None of these can affect you. Apart from your heart and brain, your stomach is the most important organ of your body.

I have known many patients – quite a few of whom were part of the clinical trials of our herbal drugs – suffering from cysts, fibroids, ulcers, tumours and cancers. All of the female patients had one thing in common: they all had sensitive stomachs and frequently suffered from indigestion or constipation. The common factor among both the male and the female patients was that their diets had a high acidic content. I must add, while I am at it, that these people were generally soft and sensitive types and not at all rough and ready. They worried more than the average person. So, without a doubt, their mental health played an important role in their physical disorders, but poor digestion was the common denominator among them.

When undigested food stays in your stomach, metabolic processes continue to work in an attempt to break it down. Gaseous toxins mix with your blood and are transported to all parts of the body. Blood oxygen levels drop, and that presents the perfect breeding ground for cancerous cells. Every human body has cancerous cells. These are extremely active and robust cells that can grow at a pace much faster than normal cells in the body. Cancerous cells or tumours have more potential to grow in areas where there is a congregation of nerves, because such plexuses of nerves suffer the most from a lack of oxygen. Breast cancer, brain tumours, ovarian cysts and fibroids are most common in women with poor digestion. A weak stomach for men may lead to prostate cancer and brain tumours.

Modern science mostly disagrees with the above analysis, but the yogic belief is quite straightforward: shallow breathing and poor digestion create a toxic environment in our bodies. It means greater retention of carbon dioxide and reduced oxygen supply. Lumps, cysts, tumours and cancerous cells thrive in such environments.

If pitta is vitiated on top of a weak digestion, it can lead to pancreatic cancer. Furthermore, cancerous cells and tumours (benign or malignant) are anaerobic: they do not need oxygen supply to grow. In fact, they are killed if oxygen is flushed through the body's internal transport system. In the chapter 'Physical Cleansing' (Chapter 13), I discuss the methods of strengthening your digestion. For those with the tendency to have lumps and cysts, deep breathing alone can do miracles, because it is capable of supplying your blood with excess oxygen.

I have seen remarkable results from deep breathing with cancer patients. Deep breathing is highly detoxifying. This is covered in more detail in Chapter 15 on 'Mental Detoxification'. For now, just understand this: if your digestion is poor, you need to attend to it now if you want to lead a healthy life. Hypertension (blood pressure), stiff joints and body aches – they all spring from poor digestion. A clean and healthy colon is the fountain of youth and vitality.

SUGAR

Even if your digestion is strong and there is little or no ama, excess sugar intake is bound to make you sick. Even five thousand years ago, sugar was a challenge for Ayurvedic physicians. The challenge then was much more manageable, though, because only handmade drinks and sweets contained added or excessive sugar. Most of the other ingredients in those times were purely natural and if they contained any sugar (carbohydrates), they contained good sugar – it had dietary fibre as well as other groups of nutrients. This is not the case today.

Today, you can consume carbohydrates with absolutely no nutritional value. For example, soft drinks, energy drinks, white flour and processed food have excessive carbohydrates and are practically devoid of nutrition. When I was an asthmatic child, my Ayurvedic physician gave me a long list of things not to eat. Potatoes, sugar, milk, chocolates, sweetmeats, soft drinks, white bread and white rice were banned from my diet. Every time I broke the rules, I paid the price – I ended up in the hospital that night. If you examine the list above, excepting milk, all these foods are rich in sugar with practically no other nutrition in them.

Almost all inflammatory diseases in the body are caused by sugar. They include, but are not limited to, asthma, allergies and sensitivities, bronchitis, oedema, eczema, rheumatoid arthritis, inflammation in the bladder or prostate, hay fever, periodontitis (inflammatory diseases affecting the gums and tissues that support the teeth), atherosclerosis (thickening of the arterial walls), inflammatory bowel diseases and many autoimmune diseases (arising from an inappropriate immune response from the body against substances and tissues present in the body). Obese people in particular have been noticed to have chronic inflammation due to raised levels of insulin, blood glucose and leptin (a protein that regulates how much fat is stored in the body), among other markers. Changes in blood glucose levels directly impact metabolic homeostasis. It vitiates the three doshas and impairs – even deludes – the immune system of the human body.

If you want to live longer and healthier, one of the first tangible steps to take is to cut down on your sugar intake. Almost all foods we consume contain sufficient natural sugar. You don't need to consume additional sugar; it will only cause harm. All artificial sweeteners are little doses of poison. There are two key hormones you should know about – both are pancreatic hormones: insulin and glucagon. Insulin gets rid of the excess sugar and glucagon supplies it when it is needed. Between the two of them, they maintain a careful balance of blood sugar levels in your body.

This is how insulin works: any excess sugar in your blood is converted into glycogen in the liver and is supplied to the muscle and adipose tissue to reduce the blood sugar level. If you don't burn this excess sugar supplied to your muscles and fat cells by exercising, it is eventually converted into body fat. When you have long gaps between your meals, your body starts to release glucagon to increase the blood sugar level to give you the necessary energy for survival. If you eat food while the blood sugar level is on the rise, suddenly your body ends up with excess sugar because there is sugar (carbohydrates) in the food too.

While the insulin is doing its work, the kidneys retain salt. To maintain the sodium levels, the kidneys dilute the salt by retaining more water. This results in more blood in the body that requires more pumping, which causes high blood pressure. Sugar also hardens the walls of the arteries and makes them narrow. Remember caramelized sugar or plain sugar candies? That's how hard sugar can get. Narrower arteries require the heart to pump harder to circulate the blood.

All starchy foods, all sugary drinks and many processed and canned foods are full of sugar. White rice, white bread, white flour, breakfast cereals and cakes and muffins also have a lot of sugar in them. Fruits are full of sugar too; their intake should be regulated. But they are also packed with the goodness of vitamins and enzymes, so you should have them. But unless you burn the excess sugar, any type of carbohydrate will harm you. In olden times, lifestyles were not so sedentary: people ate everything and physical work burnt any excess carbohydrates, so they remained healthy. Our modern lifestyles are very different though.

STRESS

Our race was never designed to handle the self-created stresses of the contemporary world. Nature did not create the stock markets, world governments or political boundaries. It did not invent the concept of large corporations and ridiculous targets. It did not evolve to create socially isolated individuals glued to a screen. It only created giant mountains and green meadows, the blue sky, pristine rivers, the vast ocean, countless beautiful and fragrant flowers and millions of species. It created the perfect ecosystem to ensure the healthiest survival of all its creatures. There were really no diseases. Either you lived healthily or you fell victim to a predator or a calamity. To fulfil its goal of a flawless operating model – to ensure the survival of species – it created a standard response system to any life-threatening situation. It was fight, flight or freeze.

Whenever any event or situation threatened one's existence, it created great stress in the brain that would trigger a whole heap of chemicals, hormones and adjustments in the body. It would hyper-activate the sympathetic nervous system. As a result, the heart would beat faster, blood flow to the skeletal muscles would rise, and the blood pressure and respiration rate would go up. To best prepare the body for a fight or flight response, the brain would reduce blood flow to the skin and gastrointestinal tract. Such an increase in the strength and agility of the limbs was compensated for by the slowing down of intestinal movement, directly affecting digestion and endocrinal secretions. The body would become tense, the heartbeat would rise – pumping more blood and oxygen in the legs – because the brain thought that digestion of food could be delayed, since the creature might need to run to save its life.

Whenever we perceived any threat, our brains began preparing our bodies for survival, completely disrupting and adversely affecting their normal functioning. The chemicals they released in the process were used to help us fight or flee. Not bad, but of much less use today.

Our stresses in the modern world are usually not real. They don't require a release of chemicals. When a company is downsizing or when the markets are crashing, we are not expected to get up from our desks, run across the street and climb up trees. We are expected to sit there and drink more caffeine and absorb the situation. The problem is that we know this, but our brains don't. They haven't yet evolved enough to differentiate between real and fake stress signals. They don't know that you wish to handle your corporate financial crisis by raising more capital, and not your heartbeat; by being calm and not distressed. Our mammalian brains continue to release chemicals at any stress signal, and when they are not used, they wreak havoc on our bodies – most notably on our digestion.

Stress is the greatest and deadliest of all diseases. If indigestion is the only physical disease, stress is the only mental disease. They fuel each other; stress almost instantly weakens your digestion. When you are stressed, your brain sends a signal to the pancreas and other glands to release additional sugar into your body. Obeying the command, your pancreatic and adrenal glands secrete glucagon and adrenaline respectively. Since it is a fake signal, insulin swings into action to get rid of the excess sugar, sending it to your muscle and fat cells. But they have no need for it either, and it may convert into body fat. This leads to high blood pressure; it is directly linked to heart disease and indigestion. Stress immediately vitiates the three doshas and is considered a tamasic (mode of ignorance) response.

This must be emphasized: stress is not a mental affliction but a response. You have no control over the stock markets, economy, governments, global problems, or a highway traffic jam, but you have control over the response you choose in any adverse or undesirable situation. Prolonged stress can, and often does, lead to depression. Most chronic ailments cannot develop in just a weak body alone; there must be an unsound mind too, because for any disease to be chronic, your body must consistently provide the environment for it to thrive.

Having chronic ailments means that the immune system isn't strong enough; that your body is not able to heal itself. More often than not, this happens because an ailing mind impairs and obstructs the normal functioning of the body. When you are stressed, your body does not produce growth hormones because it is already flooded with adrenaline and cortisol (a type of hormone). This has a telling impact on your physical health. Sound sleep, without the aid of pills or intoxicants, is a distant dream for one who is mostly stressed. And a stressed person is also highly likely to suffer from indigestion.

Stress, being a response, often becomes a habit. Those who tend to get stressed can freak out at the smallest of incidents. They can get stressed about organizational changes, about traffic on a highway, about rising gold prices and falling markets – even if they have no investment in the markets. They could get stressed if their child comes home late or if their computer crashes. When stress becomes your coping mechanism for every unpredictable situation, you lose control of yourself and the situation. You can almost be certain that ailments like diabetes, hypertension and heart problems are waiting just around the corner.

In olden times, there was a community support structure; people lived in larger families. While this arrangement had its own challenges, it allowed people to cope better with stress. There was someone to talk to; there was an outlet. Research has shown repeatedly that social isolation magnifies stress.

A pertinent question is: can you lead a life free of stress? Well, things will continue to happen around you; there are always going to be worries. But, yes, you can choose to not let them stress you out. Feeling a momentary sense of stress is natural, even instinctive, and doesn't do damage. But harbouring it is neither natural nor instinctive. It is a habit. In this, you need to remind yourself that the world does not end here and that your present response is doing you great harm.

Playing your favourite sport or engaging in an activity you love can be a great de-stressor. For example, playing a musical instrument, painting, meditation, dancing, playing sports and going to the temple or church can help you take your mind off worries and calm you down. To stop the adrenaline rush that comes from stress, your mind must return to a state of calm. Normally, distractions weaken your resolve and concentration, but in the case of stress, distractions can be real friends. Distract your mind or focus it elsewhere. There are additional methods you can adopt. I cover them in Chapter 15 on 'Mental Detoxification'.

If you eat alkaline foods, regulate your sugar intake and learn to manage stress, you can almost be assured of good health and longevity. This is the essence of all the classical and modern texts on health and wellness. You now understand the concept of constitution, the nature of food, the eating sense and the origin of diseases.

Mental Afflictions

Why do we behave the way we do? Why do we feel angry or upset? What creates fear in us, or more importantly, why do we react in a fearful manner?

Yogic and Vedic texts frequently use a term called vritti. There is no real equivalent word in the English language, but the words 'tendency' and 'temperament' come quite close. Vritti refers to the fact that each of us is born with certain tendencies. The literal meaning of vritti would be mode of life or mode of conduct. The vritti of a cow is to be gentle and quiet, of a tiger to pounce. The vritti of a snake is to attack in defence, and for a sparrow to fly away. Our vrittis make us behave a certain way.

More importantly, vritti is derived from the root element vri, meaning screen or veil. Hiding behind our vrittis is the real us: our true nature of love, compassion and eternal bliss. Since our vrittis make us behave a certain way, we start to label each other according to our feelings and tendencies. 'She is an angry woman', for example, or 'he's a jealous man'. The truth is that she is not angry and he's not jealous by birth. These emotions are simply hiding who they really are. This is why the same person can be very loving or very angry. Vrittis are like the waves in the ocean – constant and kinetic.

Our vrittis propel us to lead our lives the way we do. They make us passionate about one pursuit and indifferent towards another. Out of the many vrittis, there are some that undermine our physical and mental health. These are the prajna-aparadha (intellectual transgressions) as elucidated earlier. It means there are certain responses we choose consciously that have a negative impact on us. These responses are called mental afflictions.

The mental afflictions expounded here are emotions or emotional responses that vitiate the three doshas. Almost invariably, they lead to hypertension, diabetes, heart disease and gastrointestinal disorders. Emotions and our stomachs are inextricably related. The first part of the physical body to receive the effect of any emotion is the stomach, followed by the heart and the brain. There are five primary mental afflictions that are detrimental to one's physical, mental and emotional equilibrium.

FEAR

Any creature born with consciousness has fear, both instinctive and conditioned. Instinctive fear is what we are born with and conditioned fear is what we acquire. A shudder in the body at a sudden loud noise is instinctive fear, for example. The thought that I'll suffer in hell if I steal or do bad karma is conditioned fear. Fear can make us angry, greedy, insecure, negative, pessimistic, hateful or all of these. Whether it is the fear of rejection, of failure, of loss or of death, it can make you do impossible things –

either negative or positive. Fear weakens you; it impairs your ability to think clearly. Any threat – perceived or real – triggers a range of chemical reactions in your body, adversely affecting your well-being. Fear is always born of anticipation. There is no fear in the present moment. It is when you start to wonder what may happen in the future – immediate or distant – that you sow the seed of fear in your consciousness.

Fear immediately vitiates the three doshas and upsets your physical and mental equipoise. An asthmatic patient may get an asthma attack in fear and a patient of depression may get a panic attack, for example. It brings to the fore any underlying disorders and makes them worse in the longer run. It stops us from being positive and happy.

When you no longer feel positive about your actions or goals because you are afraid that life may just go to jelly on you, remind yourself of all the times in the past when you felt the same, but each time your fears were proven unfounded. Fear makes us feel that this is the end of the world, but the world is eternal and your world is always moving. When companies were downsizing, the economy was in depression and the stock markets were going south, you might have been affected. But you moved on.

There is only one antidote for fear, and that is action. Action directed at the cause of fear alone dispels it. Thinking about it or artificially consoling yourself will do you no good. If your fear is grounded – that is, you have a real reason to be afraid – the only way to get rid of it is to work towards it.

Imagine a heart attack survivor who has already undergone major surgery. He's afraid that a heart attack may be fatal the next time. If he consumes food that is harmful to him but mentally consoles himself, thinking that he'll be okay, the truth is that he won't be okay. Artificial consolation is not going to help him. If he's serious, his actions must support elimination of fear. On the other hand, there may be another, similar patient, who is eating well but is still worried about death or another heart attack. In this case, he needs to learn to drop his fears. Fear begins from a thought. If we can drop the thought, fear goes away too.

ANGER

The chemical reaction in the brain is almost identical in instances of anger and fear. In both cases, the brain starts to prepare a fight-or-flight response born of a need to protect against the wrong being committed or the danger. Grinding of the teeth, flushing, prickly sensations, paling, fist or jaw clenching, sweating and increased heartbeat are common reactions in anger. Anger, however, is not just a response but an emotion.

Anger can be so ingrained in some that they are completely unaware of it. How you experience and express your anger is often dependent on your emotional set-up, your psychological make-up and your upbringing. Other factors such as your environment at home and outside and conditioning by your culture and religion greatly influence how you deal with anger. Some hold on to it and many express it fully. Both are damaging, though. While fully expressing anger may cost you relationships, holding on to anger is just as big a blunder. Anger is primarily of two types.

Reactive Anger

Reactive anger can be your emotional, physical or psychical response to an unmanageable situation. It could be your impulsive response, triggered by sadness, disgust, surprise or fear. If it is simply a reaction – an outburst – you may even feel lighter and better afterwards. This is often an illusion, though. Expressing anger to feel a sense of relief becomes your standard coping mechanism in all undesirable situations.

When anger is caused by sadness, it may be a release of clogged-up negativity and frustration. When it is due to disgust, fear or surprise, however, it is your spontaneous response; it is like someone catching you off-guard, and it is more like a fit of rage. You may feel like breaking things, kicking, punching and screaming. It is rather common for people to shout when anger is a matter of reaction.

Reactive anger is like a volcano. Some people erupt under pressure. Others pop like an inflated balloon when pricked by adversities. They express their anger by way of an emotional outburst or by a fit of rage, almost hysterically. People in rage are beside themselves in no time and then they calm down. Often, they repent their actions later: they may even apologize and vow to not get angry again. All this proves futile.

The next time they experience any friction or opposition, they behave in exactly the same manner. This is mostly because an outburst of anger has become their escape route, a way of dealing with difficult situations — for as long as their own body can endure it. Just as they feel happy in desirable situations, they feel angry in all undesirable situations.

Toxic Anger

When you suppress any emotion, it settles in your consciousness like a poisonous seed. With more suppression over a period of time, it thrives and grows, eventually causing enormous, sometimes irreparable, damage to your body and mind. When you are unable to express or let go of negativity and hurt, and you keep it within you, it becomes increasingly toxic over a period of time, often leading to depression and anxiety. It can bring damning metabolic changes, resulting in severe headaches and weight gain. It can trigger heart disease, high blood pressure and cancer. Yogic and Ayurvedic texts state that anger and other negative emotions have a direct negative impact on the quantity of prana vayu, the vital life force in the air we inhale. And a lack of prana causes tumours, among other metabolic, hormonal and glandular disorders.

Toxic anger is like brewing coffee. Beyond a certain point, it gets bitter, way too bitter to be consumed; it cannot be sweetened with honey any more. Similarly, when a person holds on to his negative emotions, this negativity keeps on brewing, only making the person more bitter. Brewing anger can easily lead to a fit of rage, because an outburst is more a symptom than a cause; it is a sign that you have been holding on to negative emotions within you. It is like heating up a steamed dumpling in a microwave oven. The dumpling is able to take heat to a certain degree, beyond which it simply explodes, splattering everywhere; it is then no longer edible, much less presentable.

The more attached you are, the greater your anger. Vedic texts list both attachment and anger as mental afflictions. The extent of hurt you experience is directly proportional to the degree of attachment you have. For example, if you are really attached to your possessions, whenever something goes wrong with them, you are likely to experience grief. The greater the attachment, the more the grief, and in turn, the greater the pain – and anger follows in tow. Above all, anger is a symptom of your inner pain. It means you are hurt somewhere within; the grief is still there.

I am a monk and I meet thousands of people. Often, I find that people are too hard on themselves. They are under a huge burden of mostly unrealistic expectations. It is important to live your life with a sense of freedom. The more you do that, the less you are frustrated, and less frustration means much less anger.

Anger is a force. It is a form of energy. Therefore, like any other energy, it can be channelled and transformed. Direct it towards empathy and forgiveness and it transforms into love and compassion.

HATRED

There is a word called dvesha in Sanskrit. It is made from the union of two words: da + visha. Among other things, da means a mountain and visha means poison. Hatred is a mountain of poison. A pinch is enough to kill someone: imagine what a mountain would do! In the case of material poison, it kills a person once, but hatred is a poison that kills every moment, with every breath, with every thought. People can hate other religions, political parties, other people, countries, their loved ones, their friends and family. The object of hate becomes immaterial, because hatred is simply a misdirected emotion. The one who has hatred for one thing will always find his hatred shifting from one thing to another. Whom or what he hates is insignificant; the truth is that hatred is an emotion, an attitude, a response – even a state of mind.

Just like attachment, hatred is often an obsession too. Hatred is a deadly mental affliction. It has the same effect as toxic anger mixed with stress. Mostly, it sits in the silent corner of one's heart. Its basis could be one's experiences in the world or simply mental conditioning. Society, religion and culture – they all condition you. You are told what is good and bad, moral and immoral, right and wrong and acceptable and unacceptable.

For example, in certain sects of Hinduism, you are taught that slaughtering animals and eating non-vegetarian food is immoral. If you are a Christian, it is acceptable. If you are a Muslim, it's okay only if the meat is halal, and if you are a Jew, only if it is kosher. The environments at home and outside – and especially religion – give you a set of rules; some spoken and some unspoken. Whenever you see anyone transgressing your framework of rules, you experience hatred, however subtle it may be. Hatred creates the division of 'us' and 'them'. Hatred does not stand on its own, though. Anger and lack of understanding are the two feet of hatred.

Anger fuels hatred. When you are angry and you are hateful towards something or someone, your anger rises along with your hate. Your peace of mind is robbed. Unfortunately, the object of your hatred is often unaware of your feelings, so it rarely ever solves any purpose. Hatred in relationships could arise from untoward experiences you might have gone through, or it could be because your expectations have been mismanaged.

For example, let's say a child's parents are divorced and the father gets custody of the daughter. The father remarries and his new wife does not treat the child well. The father is busy at work; he is preoccupied enjoying his new relationship and is unable to pay as much attention to his daughter as before. The daughter feels betrayed. She has certain expectations from her father, and some from her stepmother too, but they are crushed.

As she sees her stepmother get closer to her father, she feels more out of place, even helpless. She experiences anger but is not always able to express it. This suppression of anger, along with the shattering of her expectations, clouds her understanding. She starts to see either her father or her stepmother as the cause of her negative feelings. When her understanding is clouded, hatred germinates in her mind. She may also begin to hate her mother, thinking she didn't do her job properly and that she could have avoided the divorce. Thus evolves the chain of hatred.

At the core of hatred is the absence of understanding of the other party's perspective. I have observed, on countless occasions, that it is not that people are unable to understand or appreciate a different viewpoint, they often just don't want to. The comfort zone in one's own negative and positive emotions, and in one's own belief system, can make one completely dull. The more widely travelled you are or the more exposed you are to the world and its whims and variances, the more likely it is that your understanding will be deepened. Travel and good reading does that – it opens you up. Just like butter melts in the heat, the warmth of knowledge can easily melt one's hatred.

In relationships, when you start to see that everyone is simply a medium – that you have to take responsibility for your own actions, for your own life – you start to see things differently. No doubt life may have been hard on you. Perhaps your partner, your friends, this world, your parents or your siblings may not be the best. But the truth is that ultimately you have to take charge of your own physical, mental and emotional state. Because when you are down and when you are hurt, others continue to lead their lives in the manner they see fit. Your mental afflictions are going to hurt you the most.

For your own good and well-being, it is important to be free and light. The greater your burden of various negative emotions and expectations, the weaker your body and your mind become. In a burdened mental state, you can take the best herbs, the best diet, or you can do the best workouts, but they will do little to save you from the onslaught of various physical and mental ailments. When you start to see the other person's perspective – when you develop understanding – your hatred will either turn into compassion or indifference. While compassion is better than indifference, they both make you strong.

Hatred is such a closed, aggressive and aggrieved state of mind that it completely wrecks your equilibrium. If there is an emotional or mental equivalent of cancer, it is hatred. It vitiates the three doshas and upsets the seven dhatus, the ten energies, and the five fires. You must tread the path of forgiveness, compassion and wisdom to transform this emotion into love. You cannot hate what you understand. The methods contained in Chapter 15 'Mental Detoxification' can help you cleanse and purify yourself.

JEALOUSY

This is the third mental affliction. But in no way is it any less damaging than the others. It is called matsara in Ayurvedic and yogic texts. Interestingly, the word matsara is derived from the root word mada which means intoxicating. This offers us two valuable insights. Just like an intoxicated person has lost the sense of discrimination and coordination, a jealous person too can no longer differentiate right from wrong. There is a mismatch between their actual physical actions and what they would like to do.

The other insight is that jealousy is a toxic emotion. It is intoxicating, because it poisons the mind of the one who is jealous. It is an expensive emotion. It costs us our peace and happiness. Perhaps of all the fundamental negative human emotions, jealousy would top the list. No matter how rich or poor you are, how healthy or unwell you are, how beautiful or ugly you may be, how well loved or rejected you may be, you can be afflicted with jealousy. It almost seems that jealousy has no basis. Even the most stable people can be struck by jealousy.

Jealousy is a paradoxical emotion. You are jealous when you think you deserve what another person has. But at the same time, you subconsciously believe you are not as good as the other person, and that is why he has what you want. The truth is, superiority has nothing to do with the feeling. It is simply about attitude and perspective.

At the core of jealousy and envy is comparison, but there is a slight difference between the two. In jealousy, there is always another contender. You may be envious of someone or his circumstances, but generally you are actually jealous of someone. In envy, one thinks: 'How well off so-and-so is' or 'I wish I could have that'. In envy, you don't necessarily want the other person to be deprived of what he has; it's just that you desire that too. Simply put, jealousy always involves at least three people, including you and the two people who have incited that jealousy, whereas envy may have only two people all up.

Envy may even propel you to take positive action. Jealousy is an altogether different emotion. You feel the other person is taking away something that should belong to you, so you covet what he has. It is not a win-win situation – it can't be. For you to be happy, the other person will need to part with what he wishes to keep.

Jealousy can easily trigger hatred or anger or both. What makes jealousy so pervasive is that it can be borne either out of love or hatred. No other emotion exists so gloriously and effortlessly among both the negative and positive emotions. Regardless of how you look upon jealousy or what causes it, the truth is that it is a destructive emotion and once again, like the other mental afflictions, it vitiates the three doshas and other vital aspects of your health.

A thing to remember about mental afflictions is that they are very hungry. Always. The more you feed them, the stronger they become. When you can't get rid of your negative emotions, they become the consumers of your physical and mental food. Any nutrition you provide your body is consumed by negative emotions; only the residue – devoid of nourishment – is left for you. You may take medication, supplements and eat a good diet – these are all consumed by your jealousy and anger. Only the toxic residue becomes the basic building material of your body. The same is true for your mental food too. Thoughts and emotions are food for the mind. When you are gripped by jealousy, all of your positivity and positive emotions are consumed by it.

GREED

Greed is a highly overpowering emotion. When overcome by greed, a person is willing to do anything and justify all of his actions, right and wrong, without any sense of remorse or guilt. Greed is a kinetic emotion; it carries tremendous momentum. When directed positively, it may manifest as ambition, but when it's negative, it is nothing but purely destructive. The basis of greed is dissatisfaction or discontentment. With ambition, you are grateful for what you have and you proceed to obtain more with a sense of positivity, often treading the right path. In greed, however, you are not grateful for your present situation. No matter how much you have, it always appears insufficient. It is a blind and depressing emotion.

The Sanskrit term for greed is lobha. It doesn't just mean greed, though. Lobha also means perplexity and confusion – it means impatience, temptation and eager desire as well. In Vedic scriptures, lobha is the offspring of deceit (dambha) and illusion (maya). This is what sets greed apart from ambition or mere craving. Greed is an inherently negative emotion that arises from uncontrolled temptation and a loss of wisdom. When one is prepared to use deceit to satiate a temptation, this is inevitably greed.

It is the seed of the mother of all negative emotions – fear. Fear is the greatest mental affliction. It causes the greatest insecurity. Greed propels you to engage in misdeeds, and that creates fear in the mind – fear of shame or fear of being exposed. Now, you have to conceal your acts. This may require lying or distorting the truth. It is a chain reaction. Stress, anger and fear dominate, and from the perspective of health, it's only downhill now. This saps your mental energy, causing weakening of the appetite, creating disequilibrium and completely destroying your peace and calm.

People who suffer from these mental afflictions find it hard to stand themselves, so they resort to excessive socializing or drinking to forget themselves. They can't go to sleep unless they have a drink or a sleeping pill. Diet or food alone can never make you lose your sleep. The chances are, it's one of the above five afflictions or a guilty conscience that is consuming you.

Fortunately, these emotions are not permanent. It is possible to eliminate them from your system. The path is simple. Your physical health promotes your mental well-being and your mental health supports your physical wellness. Besides the right diet and mindful living, there are other steps you can take to enjoy fine health. I am dividing those steps into two parts: Physical Cleansing and Mental Detoxification.

Physical Cleansing

Hamish and Irene, who lived in the US, had been married for nearly seven years. Hamish was a first-generation immigrant from India and Irene was of Japanese descent, born and raised in the United States. They owned three convenience stores, had no personal debt and shared a healthy relationship. Not everything was well, though. Irene was in her mid-thirties and had been desperately trying to conceive for five years. With each passing day, and with each failed treatment, the couple's despair built. They went to the best specialists and took all sorts of medication, but to no avail. The medicines and stress caused havoc in Irene's body. In the preceding three years, she had become a patient of thyroid dysfunction and hypertension and had gained twenty pounds in weight.

Medically, there was absolutely nothing wrong with either of them. All their reports were fine. They tried Ayurvedic, homeopathic, Greek, Chinese, and other oriental systems of medicine with no result. They had healthy lifestyles, which included exercising, healthy eating and the occasional consumption of seafood, chicken and red meat. None of this I considered unhealthy, given their genetic disposition and cultural backgrounds. Her inability to conceive a child, however, was having a negative impact on their relationship.

In their moments of intimacy, no love was present: it had become simply an act, an attempt to conceive. Irene started living by the calendar so that she could have the most sex during the days she was ovulating in order to conceive. This put Hamish off, but he carried on because he wanted a child as much as she did.

Hamish had known me since his days in India. Over the years, we had lost contact, as I had moved to Australia when he was still in India. Through a friend of a friend, he traced me and broke down during the very first phone call. He wasn't as concerned about having a family as he was about Irene and their relationship. He asked me if there was any hope for them, whether they could do anything astrologically, or medically, if there was any healing I could do, or if I could give them any amulet or talisman or any tantric remedy.

I was due to fly out to San Jose two weeks after we spoke. Hamish and Irene agreed to meet me there. I had met many childless couples, but Irene's desperation was not ordinary. What had aggravated it were the taunts from her in-laws that she was a 'defective piece'; that because she belonged to a different culture and caste, she was not fit to bear Hamish's child. Irene's parents were of little help as well, since they had been against the marriage from the beginning – they were both doctors, whereas Hamish was a simple convenience store owner.

Hamish even thought that some relatives of his had practised black magic on him out of jealousy, because he had 'made it' in the US. From being an immigrant with just a few hundred dollars, he had built a business of three convenience stores and had a net worth of more than a million dollars. Irene was starting to believe him too; both were searching for answers in anything. Needless to say, I didn't believe in their explanations of black magic or the evil eye, nor did I plan to give them a talisman or a meditation. I didn't even want to change their diet. I tried a different approach. The question that went to the heart of the matter was why Irene couldn't conceive if nothing was medically wrong with them.

As far as I was concerned, medication was no longer an option. According to Ayurveda, if a medicine can't cure you in nine months, it cannot cure you. Nine months is enough time for a medicine to effect a change in the whole body, because new skin is formed, new cells are created and new blood is formed within this period. If a system of medicine fails to cure in nine months, one should look for alternatives. Hamish and Irene had already been through the alternatives as well. The problem was not in the reproductive fluids but in the vessel that had to hold them. Imagine a high-voltage wire that's rusty. A rusty wire is a poor conductor of electricity. Similarly, Irene's body was an inadequate conductor of the energy required to conceive and sustain a pregnancy. A thorough cleansing of her body was needed, I felt.

I advised Hamish and Irene to check into an Ayurvedic treatment centre where various cleansing and rejuvenating treatments were to be given to their bodies over a period of a few weeks. They both flew to south India and spent a month in an Ayurvedic spa. Their medicines, phones and laptops were taken from them upon entry and were only returned when they departed a month later. They were both sceptical. Irene was even concerned, because they had taken away her inhalers and her medicine for thyroid and blood pressure.

A mere two months later, Irene conceived and gave birth to a healthy daughter in due course. Even more remarkably, a few weeks after her pregnancy, she began losing the excess weight she had gained from years of medication and stress. Three years later, she gave birth to another child, a healthy boy.

Ayurveda understood five thousand years ago that the body is a vessel. It must be clean to protect its substance. Imagine putting fresh milk in an old, unwashed jug. It'll sour quickly. Even a few drops of old milk in the jug has enough bacteria to spoil the new milk. The jug needs to be washed. Along with the right food at the right time, Ayurveda describes in great detail various methods of cleansing the body. If your body is clean and if your food is clean, you will probably never need to take medicine.

Your body has a vascular system, a digestive system, a respiratory system and a cardiac system. Whether you are sleeping or conscious, it is always working. Physical cleansing comprises a set of Ayurvedic and yogic exercises to keep your system squeaky clean and free of obstructions. It is a method of detoxification. These exercises strengthen the vital energy channels, your gastrointestinal system and the seven dhatus. Some of the exercises should be done at the change of every season, some once every quarter, and some can be done monthly, weekly or even daily. Some of them require the presence of an expert to guide you in the beginning.

Let me elaborate on the various practices. Before I

do that, however, I must spell out a word of caution – a warning, in fact. Please consult your physician regarding the suitability of the following exercises for you. Most notably, some of the cleansing exercises use salt, and are therefore not suitable for hypertensive patients or those with an impaired renal function. Even borderline renal function patients, especially diabetics who may not be aware of their renal status, should not perform these cleansing exercises.

COLON THERAPY

I must start this exposition on physical cleansing with the process of cleansing your gastrointestinal tract. A clean digestive system pacifies the three doshas, makes the skin lustrous and radiant, rejuvenates you and makes you feel light. In most people's digestive tracts, particles of undigested food stick to the walls of the intestine. In the large intestine, there may be remnants of old and hardened stools. These undigested particles and un-excreted stools are highly toxic. They sit there, creating gastrointestinal problems, causing difficult bowel movements and preparing the perfect breeding ground for major chronic ailments. There are primarily two types of colon therapy in Ayurveda: conch cleansing and enema. One clears your entire gastrointestinal system and the other clears only the large intestine. You can do both at your home; neither requires any expert supervision or medication.

Conch Cleansing

The term conch cleansing is derived from the Sanskrit shankha-prakshalana. Shankha means conch and prakshalana means cleansing or bathing. If you observe a conch you can blow like a horn, you'll see a hole at the top. If you pour water in this hole, it travels through the conch and comes out from the bottom outlet. In doing so, it cleanses the conch from the inside. In conch cleansing, this is exactly what you do to your body. You cleanse the colon so thoroughly that by the end of the therapy when you drink a glass of water, you almost immediately pass water through the rectum. When you drink water and pass water for your stool – almost as clear as the water you drank – you can well imagine how clear and clean your colon must be.

How to Do It

Take about four litres of warm water. The water should not be hot, just warm – more than lukewarm but less than hot. It should be easily drinkable. In the four litres of water, put three teaspoonfuls of salt. You can reduce or increase the quantity of salt. The saltiness in the water should be as if you are drinking soup, so put salt as per your taste. Take your vessel of warm water and an empty glass, and be close to the washroom, if not in the washroom. If your washroom is large enough, you can do the whole process there; otherwise, be close to the washroom.

Drink two glasses of the salty warm water. Water with just salt alone is repulsive and you may feel like throwing up, but gently massage your belly in round circular motions and take a few deep breaths. This will help you keep the water in your stomach. It is important to not vomit the water, because this water is the cleansing agent for your digestive tract. Once you practise it a couple of times, you will not throw up. Follow the steps below for effective conch cleansing:

1. Drink two glasses of water.
2. Do some stretching. In particular, stretch your stomach. You can do so by standing straight with your legs slightly apart. Tuck your tummy in and bend a little backwards. Hold this posture for a few seconds. Go back to the original position of standing straight and relax your stomach.
3. Move your legs a little further apart now. Raise your right arm and bend to your left. This will stretch the right oblique.
4. Go back to your straight position and do this on the other side.
5. Gently massage your stomach in the natural direction of the intestine or in circular motions.
6. Drink two more glasses of water and repeat the stretching.

Most people start to feel the urge to void their bowels within the first four to six glasses of water. In case you don't, simply drink more water and do the stretching again. As you continue the process, you will start defecating almost immediately after drinking water. That's fine, that's what we want.

Initially when you do this process, the stool in the large intestine from the previous night's meal or even before – depending on the state of your digestive system – is passed. As you continue drinking the saline solution, stagnant stools start to evacuate, and you will see a change in their colour, hardness and smell. Don't stop; drink some more water and old stools that were sticking to the walls of your colon start to flush out of your system. Drink some more and soon you will be passing only brownish water. Continue the process and you will see that the water you are taking in is now coming out almost like clear water, only a little coloured. Your colon is perfectly clean now. It's clear of any mucus, undigested food particles and stagnant stools.

Any deposition on the intestinal walls is greatly cleaned. This pacifies the three doshas almost instantly. You will feel much lighter. The whole process takes between thirty and forty-five minutes depending on how clogged your colon is.

Once this is done, don't take a hot or cold shower right away. Instead, lie down on the bed for an hour and cover your head. You will feel extremely relaxed and light. You may even fall asleep but don't sleep just yet. It is important to eat something now. It's good if you have someone who can prepare food for you while you are doing the cleansing, otherwise you should prepare it beforehand so that you can feed yourself within five to ten minutes after finishing. You can take a nap after you eat something. Keeping your stomach empty after conch cleansing can cause wind. Therefore, it's important to eat something light and nutritious.

What to Eat

Just after the conch cleansing, your stomach is extremely soft and sensitive. So it is important to eat the lightest possible food with minimal dietary fibre. Your food should have proper oil in it to lubricate the walls of your intestine, and it's best to add some turmeric to it because it is antiseptic. Do not eat raw vegetables or fruits, as your intestine is quite sensitive. Eating out in a restaurant or a fast-food outlet is simply out of the question. You should have no porridge with wheat or oats in it, no cereals and no dairy (especially milk and cheese). Dairy has active bacteria and is heavy on digestion. The best food is called khichri. It's very easy to make and is very light on your digestive system. Khichri is a savoury porridge made from rice and split mung beans. It is extremely light to digest and is nutritious at the same time. In India, since time immemorial, this has been the food to serve to the old, to patients and to infants older than six months. It is detoxifying and nourishes your stomach. Here is how to cook it:

Gather the following ingredients:

Rice: ½ cup

Split mung beans (mung dal): ¼ cup.

Water: 3 cups

Ghee (clarified butter): 3 tablespoonfuls

Turmeric powder: ½ teaspoonful

Ground cumin seeds: ¼ teaspoonful

Coriander powder (optional): ¼ teaspoonful

Asafoetida powder (optional): a pinch

Salt: as per taste

It's best to separately soak the rice and the mung dal for an hour in advance. Wash the rice and the mung dal thoroughly and drain the excess water. Khichri tastes best with Indian basmati rice; its grains are thin and long and also easy on the digestion. The ghee and turmeric in the normal khichri are generally one third of the quantity stated here but in this case, we are not just cooking ordinary but medicinal khichri. You need the ghee to lubricate your intestine and the turmeric to heal and protect the soft walls of your intestine for the next little while.

On slow heat, gently warm up the ghee in a pot. After about a minute, add the ground cumin (and the coriander powder and asafoetida if you are using it). When they turn golden brown in a minute or two, add the turmeric powder. All this while, keep the heat low. Now, add the rice and mung dal. Stir the mixture thoroughly. Pour in three cups of water and sprinkle salt as per your taste.

Stir it again. Turn up the heat to no more than medium. Put the lid on the pot and let it boil slowly till both the rice grains and the mung dal are nice and soft. It may take about fifteen minutes to cook properly.

The khichri is ready. It is preferable to put additional ghee at the time of consuming it. It will prevent formation of gas.

For the next two days, it's best to eat only khichri and go on a light meal on the third day. You should strictly abstain from drinking alcohol for the next four days at least. You can eat raw vegetables and fruits starting from the sixth day.

It is normal to not pass any stool for the next twenty-four or even forty-eight hours. Don't be alarmed if this happens. Unfortunately, over the years, your stomach has got used to retaining something in it. Serious yogis ritually clean their stomach every four hours. A clean abdomen is the easiest way to remain healthy.

When to Do It

Yogic texts recommend conch cleansing at the change of every season. The seasons in India are six, not four. So, at the time this was originally documented by the sages, they recommended doing it a maximum of six times in one year. But you could do it once every quarter. It is important to take care of your diet for a few days after doing it. Conch cleansing must be done on an empty stomach in the morning. I have mentioned earlier that you should cover your head for at least an hour after you are done with the cleansing. This may seem beyond explanation, but covering your head allows you to retain body heat better and helps you regain the heat lost due to the cleansing of the colon.

It's best to rest or even sleep after having your meal. Try not to drink water before or during your meal. Doing so may create the urge to void your bowels. You can have some water after your meal if you are really thirsty. You can drink as much water as you want after a few hours, though.

Enema

This is the second colon cleansing technique. It cleanses only the large intestine, or lower belly. This is called vasti in Ayurveda. It doesn't cleanse the entire digestive tract as conch cleansing does, but it is still easy and effective. In some ways, it cleanses the large intestine more effectively than conch cleansing, because you are introducing reverse movement of the enematic fluid. Imagine cleaning a pipe in both directions, rather than cleaning it merely in one direction. This ensures better cleansing. A stool always passes in one direction, but an enema injects fluid in the reverse direction.

In Ayurveda, an enema is not just done with water. There are a variety of herbal concoctions and decoctions for this purpose, and it is even done with oil. An enema is a far better alternative to laxatives. The downside of modern laxatives is that your body gets used to them and they even cause damage to your intestine. There is a common misconception that having enemas can become a habit. Ayurveda makes no mention of this. One is free to have an enema at least once a week. For the various herbal and oil enemas, it is best to consult an Ayurvedic physician. He may recommend one for you based on your dosha. Or you can buy the standard enema kit from a drugstore. The simplest method is to do it with lukewarm water mixed with a pinch of salt.

If you follow the principles of diet and eating mentioned earlier and do conch cleansing once every quarter, you will likely not even need to have an enema, much less take laxatives. Almost all gastrointestinal disorders will have disappeared like darkness in light. No matter how healthy you are, cleansing the colon is a good practice; it'll only make you healthier.

OESOPHAGEAL CLEANSING

Airway inflammation due to allergens is normal in patients who suffer from asthma. Cleansing the oesophagus – the tubular organ proceeding from the throat to the stomach – is particularly useful for such patients. Smokers can also benefit from this cleansing. It can be done daily. It is called kunjala or dhauti in Ayurveda. This is how it is done.

Drink two glasses of lukewarm water at your usual speed – not too fast and not too slowly. Ideally, there should be some salt in the water as it ensures better cleansing, but it is not absolutely necessary. Stand a little bent with your legs apart and lower your head. Make sure your hands are clean. Now press your tongue with your index and middle fingers and slide them further into your mouth. As soon as they come close to the uvula, you will throw up. Just gently move your fingers in to-and-fro horizontal movements (towards the uvula and away from it) until you vomit all the water you just drank. This should be done in the morning on an empty stomach. Many people use a toothbrush instead of their fingers. If you gently rub the toothbrush on your tongue in the same manner as described above for your fingers, you will achieve the same outcome. Although this is designed to cleanse your passage of food, it also cleanses your small intestine in much the same way as an enema cleans the large intestine. With the reverse movement of water, your oesophagus and stomach become clean. This promotes the digestive fire and a glowing skin. The entire process takes around seven minutes.

There is another variation of dhauti that is done with a thin, almost diaphanous strip of soft cotton cloth. It is called danta-dhauti. This technique must be done under expert supervision, and therefore I will not elaborate on it here. I am simply mentioning it so that you know there is an even more rigorous method of oesophageal cleansing. It is a yogic process and even most Ayurvedic practitioners can't do it. There are numerous teachers of hatha-yoga who can teach you this if you wish. That said, the above simple dhauti is more than sufficient.

RESPIRATORY CLEANSING

Respiratory cleansing purifies your entire body. It pacifies the three doshas and strengthens the seven dhatus. It flushes your lungs and blood with fresh and abundant oxygen, boosting your immune system and improving your overall well-being. Respiratory cleansing has a calming effect on your mind as well. It improves your memory, virility (or fertility) and strengthens your neurological system. According to the yogic texts, it allows the practitioner to live longer and healthier. It is called pranayama. Prana means vital life force and yama means to elongate it. The science of pranayama is a different subject and is not part of mainstream Ayurveda.

Patanjali, in his *Yoga Sutras*, specifically states that only those who have perfected their posture should attempt pranayama. Even though it is very common in the Western world, few people understand why doing pranayama incorrectly can cause irreparable damage to your nervous system. Briefly, a true pranayama has three stages: inhalation (puraka), retention (kumbhaka) and exhalation (rechaka). Pranayama, the mother of all yogic exercises, is of twelve different types. For the purposes of respiratory cleansing, I will elaborate here three types of pseudo-pranayama; pseudo because you won't have to retain the breath, and we'll simply focus on different methods of inhalation and exhalation to cleanse and strengthen your respiratory system, nervous system and your whole body. Pranayama has a nearly instant calming effect on the mind.

Prerequisites

For all the breathing exercises, it is most rewarding to sit cross-legged. Sitting in this posture allows you better control of the flow of the vital energies in the body. In case you can't sit cross-legged, it is okay to sit in a chair. Breathing exercises should not be done while lying down. In all the exercises, your back and neck should be in one straight line. Your posture needs to be firm and straight but not tense. It is best to do these exercises on an empty stomach in the morning. If you are doing them during the day or at night, make sure there is a minimum gap of two hours between your meal and the exercise. And that's assuming you have a light vegetarian meal, because a light vegetarian meal completely digests in two hours. If you have a heavier meal, you may want to increase the gap to three hours or more.

Start all breathing exercises with an exhalation. This is a subtle but extremely significant point. Exhalation allows you to expel stale air. If you start with an inhalation, you simply pressurize toxic air, making it circulate through your system. A rule of thumb to be followed for all yogic exercises: if they make you uncomfortable, stop right away and seek expert guidance.

Simple Deep Breathing

Simple deep breathing is a hassle-free, easy and potent exercise. Assuming that you have followed the prerequisites, just sit comfortably, resting your hands in your lap if you are sitting cross-legged or on your knees if you are sitting in a chair. Inhale deeply and gently with both nostrils. Fill your belly and lungs with fresh air. Hold it for a few seconds – no more than five seconds – then exhale gently. Pull your belly in as you exhale and gently push your belly out as you inhale.

Simple deep breathing has a calming and purifying effect on your body and mind. It is the easiest of all breathing exercises and you can do it even at work. Ideally, breathing exercises should be done where you have plenty of fresh air, but even doing them indoors is better than not doing them at all. If you feel restless, agitated, irritated, fatigued or simply stressed, just do deep breathing for about five minutes and see your mental state change by the time you finish the exercise.

Set aside fifteen minutes in the morning for simple deep breathing. Do it for five minutes and take a break of two minutes and then do it for another five minutes.

Alternate Breathing

Alternate breathing is a type of pranayama that is excellent for neurological and respiratory cleansing and detoxification. It forms part of the nervous system purification (nadi-shodhana) regime. It is called anuloma-viloma in yogic texts. Anuloma means natural order and viloma means reverse order. While retention of breath is an important aspect of pranayama, it is recommended only for those who have mastered the physical posture, who eat a sattvic diet and who are complete teetotallers. You should note that the exercises in pranayama are a staged progression.

Therefore, in a variation of the standard alternate breathing, my strong recommendation is that you do not hold your breath for any more than a few seconds (between five and ten). There is a very important reason for this. When you practise alternate breathing without gaining stability in your posture and without controlling your diet, you run the risk of pushing toxins through your nervous system, to all parts of your body. This can lead to neurological disorders, the formation of tumours and cysts and loss of memory. If you practise alternate breathing without prolonged retention of breath, you gain the greatest benefit. You purify and cleanse your nervous system and boost the stabilizing energies and forces in and around you. If you have been practising yoga for a long time (a minimum of two years) and you are on a sattvic diet, you can practise breath retention for a longer time. In any case, do not do it beyond what you are comfortable with. No yogic exercise is supposed to make you red in the face, either during or after the exercise. Yogic exercises are supposed to be effortless.

To do alternate breathing, follow these instructions. As always, start by exhaling completely from both nostrils. Put the thumb of your right hand on your right nostril to close it. Now breathe deeply, steadily and gently through your left nostril. Hold the breath for a few seconds. Put the middle finger of your right hand on the left nostril and lift your thumb to open the right nostril. Exhale completely, steadily and gently. Ideally, your exhalation should be so soft that you should not even hear yourself breathing out. Yogic scriptures state the standard one-four-two rule for pranayama. It means if it takes you one second to breath in, for example, you should hold the breath for four seconds (four times the length of inhalation) and exhale over two seconds (double the length of inhalation). However, as I stated earlier, retention of breath should only be done if you are observing all the rules and if you have been guided by an expert.

If you have epilepsy or hypertension or suffer from palpitations, or if you have had a heart attack in the past, do not retain the breath at all. Simply breathe from alternate nostrils. At one stretch, you can do twenty repetitions. One complete repetition is inhale from the left, hold, exhale from the right, inhale from the right, hold, and then exhale from the left. This is one repetition. If you have the time, you are free to do it twice or even thrice a day. There is no better purifier of your entire nervous system than pranayama. It is nothing short of a miracle exercise, handed down to us by the ancient yogis.

Bellows Breathing

This is called bhastrika in yogic texts. The metaphor in the texts for this exercise is the bellows of a blacksmith's fire. But finding a blacksmith's fire these days is harder than sourcing ancient yogic manuscripts. So instead, imagine using a hand pump to inflate a tire. It has two movements:

push down and pull up. If you push down and pull up at the same speed, you are doing bhastrika. Compared to the other types of breathing exercises, this is a bit more swift and aggressive.

To begin with, just relax your body completely – especially the shoulders. Take a few deep breaths to prepare your body and stomach. Start forceful exhalations through your nose (both nostrils), immediately followed by equally forceful deep and swift inhalation. Keep your body – the torso and the limbs – as still as possible. It is diaphragmatic breathing. Only your abdomen should be seen moving. Your belly expands while you inhale and tucks towards your spine while you exhale. In other words, your body remains still and only your tummy moves in and out.

Do twenty breaths (inhalation-exhalation) in one set. Take a rest of one minute. Do normal deep breathing during the rest time and then repeat the set. You can do up to four sets. If there is a miracle to cleanse and strengthen your colon, to improve your body's metabolism and to rid yourself of most gastrointestinal disorders, then bhastrika is it. It pacifies the three doshas and gives you an amazingly healthy colon. Its results become noticeable in a matter of days.

Bellows breathing or bhastrika can be practised once or twice every day. Increase the count only steadily, preferably under guidance. Do it on an empty stomach and empty bladder. It is prohibited for pregnant women and for those with acute asthma.

SINUS CLEANSING

The nose is the body's first line of defence against any allergen. You mostly inhale and exhale through the nose –

at least you should do so – therefore, the nose responds to pollen and most other seasonal allergies first. Yogic texts place great emphasis on nasal cleansing, because besides alleviating most environmental allergies, it clears the breathing passages – a must for any serious practitioner of yogic breathing exercises. All the breathing exercises mentioned earlier are dependent on clear nasal passages.

Nasal cleansing has a marked effect on headaches, migraines and nasal polyps. It is excellent for vision and the overall health of the eyes. The exercise of sinus cleaning is called neti. The literal meaning of neti in Sanskrit is 'not this'. It is a Vedic concept of transcendental wisdom that makes the seeker aware that they are not the body, mind, senses, religion, or matter; that they are beyond the sum total of physical and perceptible aggregates. In *Hatha Yoga Pradipika*, a classical text on yoga, neti is described as the process of inserting a soft thread through your nose and pulling it out of your mouth. It may sound a bit difficult, but with practice anyone can master it in a matter of weeks, if not days. Neti is of two types: water neti and thread neti.

Water Neti

To do water neti, you will require a neti pot. These days, all major drugstores stock neti pots or you can buy them online. Put warm water mixed with salt in the pot. It is of paramount importance to put salt in the neti water, because plain water can cause the nasal turbinate to swell up, thereby worsening its condition. If you live in a region where water is highly chlorinated, you may want to boil it first. If so, filter and cool down the boiled water and use this water to do neti. Chlorinated water may be fine too, but it's better to use soft, ionized, distilled or alkalized water. Water in your neti pot should be neither too hot nor too cold. It should be on the warmer side. Pour a few drops on the back of your hand to make sure the temperature is right.

You can do it over the sink or in the shower, or anywhere for that matter where spillage of the water is not an issue. Neti can be performed standing or sitting. If you do it standing, just hold your legs apart, knees slightly bent, bend your upper body at around a seventy degree angle and lean forward a bit. If you want to do it sitting, you will need to squat. The most important thing to remember while doing neti, is to breathe only through your mouth.

Place the nozzle of the neti pot on your left nostril (you can also begin the neti through the right nostril, if you wish). Once the nozzle is snugly fitted on your nostril (you may have to turn, twist or adjust it to ensure that it completely blocks your nostril), tilt your head to your right side. Now raise the neti pot a little so that water starts to flow out from the nozzle.

It will start to pass through one nostril and out of the other. You can run half the pot through one nostril and the remaining half through the other nostril. If you feel good, you may pass one potful through each nostril. There is no hard-and-fast rule regarding this. I reiterate: make sure you remember to breathe only through your mouth while doing neti, otherwise you'll end up snorting a lot of saline water and it's not a nice feeling. It's also important to dry your nose properly once you're finished, so do soft inhalations and forceful exhalations for around a minute.

As warm water flows through your nose, it warms the sinuses and has a strange calming effect on your mind. Water neti is extremely good for sinusitis, allergies and headaches, as also for your eyes.

Thread Neti

Thread neti, or sutra neti, should only be performed under expert guidance. For informational purposes, I am documenting it here for you. Thread neti is performed either with strands of thread twisted to form a thick (around three millimetres) string or with a thin rubber catheter. Of all the yogic practices focussed on nasal cleansing, thread neti is the most powerful and effective method; water neti comes a close second. Here is how to do thread neti.

If you are using thread (as opposed to a rubber catheter), take multiple strands to form a bundle of about three millimetres in diameter and about forty-five centimetres long. Trim and twist the ends. Melt some beeswax and dip one third of the string in it. Allow it to harden. Take the other end of the string and dip one quarter in beeswax. Allow it to harden. You can also get neti threads from markets or you can simply use the rubber catheter. Personally, I use the rubber tube because it's softer and gentler on the nose. Besides, with beeswax, I can't be sure that I will get pure, organic beeswax in the market and not something mixed with chemicals. In a nutshell, a rubber catheter is simpler, economical and just as good.

Stand square with your legs slightly apart and gently insert the catheter in one of your nostrils. It'll come into your mouth and you'll feel it on your tongue. Put your index and middle fingers into your mouth, reach out to the catheter, and gently pull it out of your mouth. One end of the catheter is now hanging out of your nose and the other one from your mouth. Hold each end with your hands and gently pull to and fro a few times, then pull the catheter out of your mouth. Wash it with warm water and repeat the process on the other nostril.

Neti (water- or thread-based) opens the nasal passages and consequently you draw more oxygen into your body. It is beneficial not just for the nose but for the ears, eyes and throat as well. During the change of season, it can be done every day for a couple of weeks. Normally, it should be done no more than twice a week. It is a common practice among the yogis to put a drop of ghee (clarified unsalted butter) in each nostril after the neti to lubricate the nose. You could use some lubricating nasal drops if you do not wish to use ghee. A lot of people don't use any ghee or nasal drops. You are welcome to do what suits you best.

Fasting and Pancha-karma

We all feel good when we sleep, waking up rejuvenated and fresh. Why? Because our body and mind are able to rest when we are asleep. But our kidneys, stomach and liver are forever working. Every day we eat and all the time they are put to work. They don't get time to rest, recoup or rejuvenate.

Fasting is called vrata in Sanskrit. It means a solemn vow or a resolution. As the name suggests, fasting is a resolution to do something a certain way for a specified period of time. For example, refraining from speaking or a vow to observe silence, is called mauna vrata. Abstinence from sex is called brahmacharya vrata. Yogic and Ayurvedic texts describe many types of fasts to improve well-being.

Fasting is a powerful method of detoxification and it is not the same as starving. There is something quite subtle you should know about fasting. When you skip your meals for a whole day out of stress or due to a hectic routine, your digestive system and hormones behave in a different manner compared to when you do this as a planned fast. Therefore, skipping meals is not the same as fasting. I'll be happy if any scientist verifies this. The amount of endocrinal secretions in planned fasting is much more regulated by the brain.

Fasting, when done correctly, pacifies the three doshas, subdues inflammation and nourishes the seven dhatus. It is better to have regular and short periods of fasting. For example, let's say you go on a fast where you only consume fruit juices. Rather than fasting for one straight week on a juice-only diet, it is better to fast one day every week for the next six weeks. Prolonged fasting causes damage to the body tissues.

Fasting increases your willpower and gives your digestive system a much-needed break. Ideally, you should not fast more than one day a week. You can also choose to fast once every two weeks or once every month. You need to see what suits you based on your own constitution, your physical and mental health and your routine. Don't push yourself to fast, though – especially if you get irritated when you are hungry. There are four ways to fast.

TYPES OF FASTING

I will elaborate on the types of fasting. But first, a word of caution: please consult your physician before fasting, and specifically, patients with diabetes should not fast.

Light Fasting

In light fasting you eat a light meal only once every twenty-four hours. Remember khichri? That's a light meal. It is important to consume only one meal in twenty-four hours and nothing in between other than water. If you consume anything else in addition to this one meal, it confuses your brain and messes with the insulin regulation and hormonal balance in your body. During light fasting, it is important to either choose a savoury meal or a sweet meal. Don't go for both of these tastes. It is not prudent to have dessert after your light meal, for example, because your body then treats it as a normal meal and expects the next meal in your normal routine.

You may want to consume just the salty khichri and nothing sweet before, during or after your meal, for instance. Or you may choose to have sweet rice pudding. Not both. In light fasting, many people have their only meal before sunrise and fast for the next twenty-four hours. Some prefer to stay hungry the whole day and have their meal in the evening. Either way is fine.

Light fasting can be done once a week or once every two weeks. There are no set rules as such. Feel free to do what suits you best. During my days of intense meditation, I practised light fasting by taking only one meal every twenty-four hours for a stretch of seven months. In the first month, I ate my meal at midday, but later I started taking it before sunrise. During the day, if I needed it, I would drink upto two glasses of water. There were some days when I ate nothing but snow. This was in the Himalayas, and all my time was spent in meditation.

There was plenty of snow around then. I used to take some from the roof of my hut and eat it. It took about a week in the beginning for my body to adjust, but I felt extremely fit. My meal was conducive to my intense meditation regime. I used to put a tablespoonful of clarified butter (ghee) made from cow milk in my meal. I might add that I did mauna vrata (observing silence) and ekanta vrata (solitude) as well for one hundred days in that seven-month stretch. These have a pacifying effect on your appetite. I didn't lose any body weight compared to when I ate thrice a day. On the contrary, meditation, silence and a frugal diet gave remarkable strength to my body and mind.

Fruits-and-veggies Fasting

The primary difference between light fasting and this fast is that in fruits-and-veggies fasting, you stay off all beans and grains. Basically, you do not consume foods with gluten of any nature. A yogic diet also prohibits peas and corn. Dairy foods are permitted in fruits-and-veggies fasting, especially ghee. Ghee is a highly sattvic food and it pacifies the three doshas. It stays in the digestive tract for some time without causing indigestion and pacifies pangs of hunger that are sometimes experienced by fasters.

Ghee made from cow milk is considered better than ghee made from buffalo milk. In India, most of the ghee sold in the market is made from buffalo milk, which is richer in fat and harder to digest. In fact, in Ayurvedic preparations, when needed, only ghee from cow milk is used.

During fruits-and-veggies fasting, you are allowed to eat two portions in twenty-four hours. I once went on this fast for a stretch of thirty days. Rather than two portions, I used to eat only once in twenty-four hours, just before sunset in the evening. My diet was one glass of cow milk and one apple or one banana. It was a little hard in the beginning, but my body adjusted in a matter of a few days.

During the whole thirty days, I did not feel tired or fatigued. Nor did I feel any pangs of hunger. Although it was not my goal to lose weight, because I was already at the correct weight, I did end up losing six pounds due to the reduced intake of food. I chose this diet because I was doing a special practice of meditation that prescribed only one meal a day, with no salt, beans or grains. It may sound paradoxical, but fasting infuses the body with an inexplicable type of strength and energy.

Liquid Fasting

In liquid fasting, you do not consume any solid foods of any kind. No fruits, vegetables, grains, beans, or milk products. Some people drink milk during liquid fasting but it is not a good idea. Milk is heavy on digestion regardless of whether it is no-fat, low-fat or full-cream. A milk-only diet vitiates vata and causes gastrointestinal disorders, including constipation. If you want to go on a liquid fast, it is best to simply consume fruit and vegetable juices. Drinking just vegetable juices vitiates pitta and vata, so the consumption of fruit juice is a good idea.

With almost no fat in your diet during this fast, and your food packed with vitamins and other nutrients that are only found in fruits and vegetables, this fast is a brilliant way of detoxifying your body. If you are diabetic or on medication that requires a certain food intake, please check with your physician before undertaking this fast. Tea, coffee and alcoholic drinks are strictly prohibited with liquid fasts.

Complete Fasting

As the name suggests, you practice complete abstinence from any type of food – solid or liquid. For twenty-four hours, you feed your stomach with only your breath. Water is permitted, though. I know many people who abstain from water as well. There is a fast in India that is called nirjala vrata. It means fasting without water. It is often observed on ekadashi (the eleventh day of the lunar calendar).

People on medication should only attempt complete fasting after speaking to their physician. It is not uncommon to experience headaches or pangs of hunger. This fasting gives a complete break to your digestive and metabolic systems. According to Ayurveda, it pacifies kapha and vata in the body.

PANCHA-KARMA

Pancha-karma is the ultimate – and the most complete – detoxifying set of therapies in Ayurveda. Pancha means five and karma means therapy in this case. It pacifies the three doshas and has an amazingly calming effect on the body and mind. After pancha-karma, you feel like you are floating on air – light, rejuvenated and fresh like never before. If you have never experienced pancha-karma, I highly recommend you give it a try. It must be done by a bona fide practitioner of Ayurveda. It's not something you can do on your own.

Pancha-karma involves five treatments. In addition, two pre-purification treatments (purva karma) are done to prepare the body. Five treatments form the main treatments (pradhana karma). A proper pancha-karma takes approximately five days. The two preparatory treatments usually need to be carried out for three days. And the actual pancha-karma can be done in one day or it can be spread over two days. Many people, pressed for time or other resources, pick just one or two components of pancha-karma. Even that is better than not doing it at all. Ideally, pancha-karma should be done once every quarter at the change of a season. If you want to do it twice in a year, it's best to do it during the peaks of summer and winter. If you want to do it only once in a year, spring is the best season for this.

Preparatory Treatments

The preparatory treatments or the pre-purification therapies are divided into two parts. The first part is called snehana, or lubrication and anointing. In this treatment, you go on a specific diet – generally devoid of fat, oil and spices – for three days. Every morning, however, you are required to take a small dosage of ghee from cow milk. This is very effective in bringing all the toxins to – and lubricating – the gastrointestinal system. During the day, you take the prescribed diet. Then you are given an oil massage (abhyangama). It is a specific type of massage to soften the tissues of your body and to further move the toxins in your body to your gastrointestinal system. This is the anointing part of snehana.

It is followed by a second purificatory rite called svedana, which is sweat therapy, quite like sitting in a steam room. The toxins that have been raised to the surface of your body using oil massage are flushed out using sweat therapy. These two treatments are repeated for three days to fully prepare your body for the healing and detoxification from the pancha-karma treatment.

The five treatments of pancha-karma completely pacify the three doshas. The healing and detoxification effects stay with you for many weeks after the treatment. The five classical components of pancha-karma are as follows.

Emission Therapy

This is called vamana. It means regurgitation. After the three-day purificatory rites, you are ready to completely flush the toxins out of your system. Vamana is emission therapy, which is a form of induced vomiting. You may be given salted water or a herbal concoction depending on your constitution and condition, and then made to vomit. It is quite similar to kunjala (oesophageal cleansing) which I explained in the previous chapter, the key difference being that vamana is assisted. It is done after the pre-purification rites and, therefore, more effective.

Vamana cleanses your lungs and gets rid of mucus depositions. Ayurveda believes that suppressed emotions vitiate kapha, causing bronchitis, asthma and phlegm. The purpose of the two preparatory rites is to dislodge the mucus in your system so that it accumulates in your stomach. It is then ejected out of your system with emission therapy. Vamana is not recommended for pregnant women or old people who are in a frail condition.

Purgation Therapy

It is called virechana in Ayurveda, which means purgation. This is a medicated purgation therapy where herbs are used as laxatives. The therapy thoroughly cleanses the gastrointestinal tract. The cleansing is far more effective than normal purgation due to the use of a medicated laxative and preparatory treatments. Virechana pacifies the three doshas and is an excellent detoxifying treatment. A herbal decoction mixed in warm water is administered on an empty stomach. After the treatment, you have to be on a light diet for the following seventy-two hours.

Enema

It is called vasti or basti. This is the final step in the complete cleansing of the colon. It can be done with lukewarm salted water or a herbal preparation. In a variation, it is also done with medicated oil. Once you go through the emission, purgation and enema, your stomach is almost like an infant's. It is as clean as possible. This has a noticeably positive effect on the major disorders of the body.

Nasal Therapy

Called nasyama, in this procedure, medicated nasal drops made from oil or herbal combinations are administered. You also inhale smoke of incensing medicated herbs through your nose. Nasyama opens the nasal passages and sinuses; you experience a sudden clearing or dilation in your nose and sinuses. The snorting of smoke also brings tears to your eyes, immediately clearing the tear ducts.

There is another variation of nasal therapy called vapour nasyama. In this, you inhale the steam of a boiling herbal mixture. This reaches even further than nasal drops or smoke inhalation. Those administering nasyama to asthma patients should be particularly careful, given that asthmatics tend to be especially sensitive and not all respond well to it. It is generally followed by gargles of herbs to clean your throat, which can cause irritation.

Shiro-dhara

Shiro-dhara offers the ultimate calming experience of any treatment in Ayurveda. It has an immediate and profound effect on the central nervous system. Shiroh means head and dhara means flow. No matter how headachy you may be, or how bad your hay fever is, by the time you finish shiro-dhara, your blocked nose will be clear, your headache will be gone, and your whole body will feel light and relaxed.

In this treatment, you are made to lie down with your eyes closed and covered. Warm medicated oil is then poured on your forehead in an unbroken flow. This is done for about forty-five minutes. It is so relaxing, that many people fall asleep within the first few minutes. In a variation of shiro-dhara, rather than warm oil, cold buttermilk mixed with herbal extracts is poured on your forehead. This is called takra-dhara (where 'takra' is buttermilk mixed with a third of water), which feels like a bucket of cold water being poured on you just after a sauna. Both shiro-dhara and takra-dhara offer uniquely different experiences.

I must point out that many modern-day variations of pancha-karma – for commercial and practical purposes – do not practise vamana (vomiting) and virechana (purgation). Instead, they combine the preparatory rites with the main therapies to make five treatments. If you examine it closely, pancha-karma has similar therapies to the various cleansing exercises outlined in the previous chapter. You can do all those exercises at home. Massage and steam therapies and shiro-dhara are the only additions. If you regularly perform the cleansing exercises at home, you can simply opt for massage, steam therapy and shiro-dhara at any Ayurvedic centre. These can be done on the same day, and you'll be free within a few hours.

Mental Detoxification

Bo was a high-level executive in his mid-forties, working for a large organization. He had a happy family with a loving wife and two kids. For reasons the family did not understand, Bo was often battered by episodes of shooting pain in his right knee and wild mood swings. He was physically fit, he had no neurological disorder either. Nothing could explain his knee ache. As for the mood swings, they happened even when he was on vacation, when there was no stress of work. To make matters worse, he experienced them more in public settings. When he was in such a state, Bo often said things that hurt his wife and damaged their relationship. He would later apologize, but his apologies had little impact. His delivering her a verbal bashing and subsequently apologizing seemed like a bad, recurring pattern of intertwined behaviours.

Bo and his wife tried many things without success, until they met a brilliant therapist. He advised Bo to recall and narrate the major incidents of his life, especially those where he experienced grief and pain – physical or mental. A few hours later, they had figured out the cause of his sudden bouts of physical pain and mood swings. It turned out that while growing up, Bo was bullied in school. One particular time, a bully gave him a nasty blow on his right knee with a baseball bat. The blow did not break his knee, but the pain was excruciating, causing him to cry out aloud. He was promptly given medical aid. The bully was subsequently expelled from the school and no one ever pestered him thereafter.

This experience, however, had found a permanent home in Bo's mind. Whenever he passed through markets or shopping malls, if he saw a baseball bat or any memorabilia linked to baseball, he experienced pain in his knee. It happened in his subconscious mind; he was unaware of the link between this traumatic childhood event and his current pain. His mood swings were triggered at the sighting of anything linked to baseball, especially a bat.

Awareness of the link between his physical and emotional pain and his past trauma – along with some therapy – allowed Bo to heal himself and regain harmony within and in his marriage.

Feeling depressed, angry or constrained, or brooding are all merely the symptoms of an emotionally wounded person. They mean you are hurt somewhere within. The pain is still there even if you deny it. That is not going to help beyond a certain point. Fighting the symptoms is equally pointless.

Physical cleansing and pacifying your doshas bestows sound physical health on you. But sound physical health does not mean you will be happy and stress-free; it does not mean that you will remain eternally healthy. Our negative emotions and thoughts are toxins that cloud our thinking and sense of wellness. Therefore, in order to take your immune system to an entirely new level and to enjoy every moment of your life, so that you may actually enjoy the benefit of fine physical health, it is equally important to have a mind free of toxins.

Most people carry enormous baggage of negative and suppressed emotions, thoughts, expectations and grudges. This is often in addition to the mental afflictions I elucidated earlier. Together, these change their thinking patterns, which are at the core of automatic responses and habits. Ultimately, everything we do is to make ourselves happy and peaceful. The more purified the mind, the calmer it is going to be. Thoughts arising in a calm mind have a much better chance of manifestation than those emerging in an agitated mind.

Meditation is one of the finest methods of mental detoxification. It is the art of understanding, stilling and calming your mind. It helps you realize the full potential of your capabilities and puts you in control of your thoughts and emotions. It is not always about sitting down and building your concentration. Being conscious of your thoughts, words and actions is also meditation. For sound mental, physical and emotional health, I am sharing a few exercises with you.

VISUALIZATION FOR PHYSICAL HEALTH

It is no secret that the top athletes in the world extensively use visualization techniques as part of their mental training. Through visualization, they are able to perform better and in accordance with their own expectations. Thought is a force of energy. All the matter in the universe – and, of course, on our planet – is a form of energy. The human body is a colony of sixty trillion living cells. They have no underlying structural reality to them. At one time, scientists believed that the nucleus of an atom was a material particle, but later research and quantum physics disproved this completely. A nucleus has a proton, electron and neutron. A neutron has a quark. And neither of them have any structure; they are just a flux of energy in space.

Similarly, your body is simply a conglomerate of the tiny cells that are nothing but living manifestations of energy. With visualization, you can treat them, repair them, heal them or even kill them. During my time in the Himalayan woods, I used visualization to get rid of unbearable aches and pains in my body. Visualizations allowed me to live in the harsh Himalayan conditions on one meal a day without compromising my physical health.

You can use visualization to heal yourself; to cure chronic ailments and even to get rid of tumours in your body. The quality of the visualization has a direct influence on the degree of healing. If meditation is already a part of your daily routine, visualization can work wonders for you. On countless occasions I have used visualization to relieve my asthma and allergies. Any inflammation caused by allergens can be treated with this form of meditation. You don't have to take my word on its face value. You are free to test it and experience it for yourself.

How to Do It

Sit in the standard meditative posture. If you can't sit cross-legged, sit in a chair with your back straight. Once seated, take a few deep breaths. Imagine a certain calmness coming over you. Visualize that you are not a body made from some physical structure but trillions of cells (this is the truth anyway). Imagine these cells are white in colour and illuminating. Further, shift your attention to the ailing area of this cellular body.

Visualize that the cells in the ailing part are angry and red. They are swollen because of their negativity, and this has caused your current ailment (inflammation, clogging, swelling, cancer, a tumour or some other anomaly). Visualize calming, radiant, bluish and white waves of light pacifying these cells. Envision how they recede upon pacification and return to their original state. Imagine that they are no longer inflamed.

It may sound far-fetched, but give it a try to see its effectiveness for yourself. You can also hold a dialogue with these aggrieved cells, telling them you mean no harm and that they can relax and calm down. At the root of the last statement is a sense of compassion. These cells are living entities, micro-organisms that are part of your body but independent at the same time. If you emit thoughts of compassion for them, it works wonders. Countless times I have tried this successfully on myself, and on multiple occasions on others to help them heal quicker.

I am not suggesting that meditation is a panacea or that visualization will absolutely rid you of all ailments. But at the same time, if you do it thoroughly and regularly, there is no reason why it can't completely transform you. In Ayurveda, disease is not matter but force. In quantum physics, this universe and every material particle in it, including our own bodies, are also the mere play of forces of energy. Thought is a force too; it has energy. The proof of this is that a thinking brain consumes more energy than a sleeping brain.

The force of a visualization (which is a chain of intended and purposeful thoughts) can help you tap into the right energy cycles or alter the course of existing energy patterns in your body. The world around you has infinite energy; a thought is the only entry point into that world of energy. And meditation is the art of staying on a thought for as long as you wish.

Other than using visualization to get rid of your physical ailments, you can also use it to heal your past and the negativity stored in you. It is one of the most efficient methods for erasing your psychic imprints.

ERASING PSYCHIC IMPRINTS

Whatever we experience in life, everything we do leaves an imprint on us – a psychic imprint. These imprints conjure up our thoughts, chart our tendencies, our habits, our nature, and almost everything about us. Patanjali states in his *Yoga Sutras* that psychic imprints resulting from karma accumulate over many lives, conditioning the mind and causing us grief. The easiest way to create a new habit or get rid of an existing one is to erase the corresponding psychic imprint.

The mind's uncanny ability to store and recall thoughts in the form of images and words makes up our memory store. In your quiet moments, when you recall painful incidents, you feel indisposed. The more you try to forget them, the heavier they become; the faster you try to run away from them, the quicker they get to you. It is not possible to erase the memory per se, but it is possible to erase the impression a certain memory has left on you. Erasing the imprint or reducing its impact automatically makes the memory harmless. There are two ways of erasing those imprints: the yogic and the intellectual methods.

The Yogic Method

This method requires patience, discipline and persistence, but it's an incredibly powerful method of erasing any undesirable imprint. The success in all yogic methods depends on the aspirant's ability to sit still, concentrate and visualize. Maintaining one posture stills the primary energies; concentration stills the five secondary energies and readies your mind. The actual erasure is a process of visualization. The longer you can hold on to your visualization during your session of meditation, the quicker the healing. It is like performing surgery. You are the surgeon, your mind is the patient and visualization is the procedure. Therefore, the patient (mind) needs to be perfectly still (with a steady posture) while the surgeon (you) concentrates and does the procedure (visualization).

How to Do It

1. Sit still with your back straight, preferably cross-legged, but any other comfortable posture will do just fine for this practice.
2. Close your eyes.
3. Do deep breathing – just normal deep breathing – for a few minutes. Discriminating faculties of the conscious mind will become somewhat passive as a result.
4. Recall a person or an incident that caused you great grief in the past. Your mind will automatically pick up all related emotions and thoughts. Try, though, to stay focussed on that one person or incident.
5. Imagine releasing soft white light from your heart chakra in the form of compassion and forgiveness. Anahata chakra, known as the heart chakra, is a psychoneurotic plexus situated near your heart, in the centre of your chest – the vertical middle point between your throat and navel, between the two nipples.

If you experience guilt because you did something wrong, visualize forgiving yourself, even if you feel that you are at fault for what you had to go through. You will travel through a whole spectrum of emotions as you do this practice. Bring back your attention and focus on the calming white light. Visualize yourself being infused with it. Do not hesitate to engage in self-dialogue. Your focus, however, should not be to brood over matters but to erase and eradicate the imprint. It is not about right or wrong; it is just about forgiving for your own good. Clean the whole canvas of images. Repaint it with your favourite scene. Imagine yourself in bliss and smiling; envision living your dream, being happy, being healthy.

6. Take a few deep breaths again and slowly open your eyes.
7. If you believe in God, say your favourite prayer, or simply express your gratitude for all that you have been blessed with.

One session should last for a minimum of fifteen minutes. Be consistent. Do not expect results in the first session. Once you do this a sufficient number of times – around thirty – you will experience a miracle; you will find that recalling that incident or person no longer aggravates or irritates you. You will experience peace upon such recollection. You have successfully metamorphosed your emotion. It is a beautiful and empowering feeling.

Most yogic methods require an average of twenty-eight days of daily practice before they show any results. It takes usually six months before an aspirant starts to perfect their practice. Once you are able to practise intense visualization, you can accomplish just about anything you can imagine. Subsequent healing sessions accomplish much more, and quickly.

The Intellectual Method

Think about what happens when a child gets a new toy. He is fascinated. The more he gets to play with it, the quicker his attractions start to wither away. He gets over the toy. Earlier he would even sleep with it, talk to it, play with it; now, the toy is dead. Its sighting does not trigger any emotion in the child. Similarly –and just as naturally, albeit ironically – when you experience abuse, rejection, failure, deceit, lies and pain, your mind gets a new toy. The more you try to avoid it, the stronger the attraction. Here is an easy way to get over those emotions.

How to Do It

To carry out this practice effectively, you either need a mirror or a voice recorder. The steps:

1. Look in the mirror or turn on the voice recorder.
2. Recall a negative or painful incident from your past.
3. Start narrating it verbally, either by talking to the mirror or recording on your dictaphone.
4. Try to recall every minute detail around the incident. For example, let us assume someone you deeply loved broke up with you. The news itself was most unexpected. And the timing and manner of the break-up and the demeanour of your loved one – combined with your lack of anticipation of the event – made this a most traumatic experience. Years have passed, but you have not got over it. As part of this exercise, recall the incident. Do this boldly. Think of the colour of the walls, what you ate prior to being given the news, what all of you were wearing, what was going through your mind, how the other person looked, what objects were there in the room

and what were the surroundings. Recall all of these and speak them out.

5. Take a few deep breaths and close the session.

You will experience pain and hurt. You may experience an emotional outpouring. Be bold. Do all this multiple times over a number of sessions. Play with this toy. You can later listen to your own recording. As you do, you will recall even greater detail. Over a period of time, as you do your sessions, the whole incident – the person and that phase of your life – will cease to matter. After fifteen to twenty sessions, its impact will simply disappear. Forever.

It is paramount to recall as much detail as possible. And here is why. Remember Bo? If you do not recall the detail, you will not be able to erase the pain. If you are unable to erase it, whenever you see similar coloured walls, people with similar expressions, even food like you had that day, it will silently trigger the negative or draining emotion in you. Hence, I cannot stress enough the importance of recalling as much detail as possible. The information recall in the fifth session, for instance, will be much greater than the first. So repeat this exercise till you get over the incident completely. The devil is in the detail.

You can also do this exercise with a friend who is willing to listen to you without judgement. You could take turns. You could help the other person heal, and they could help heal you. That is why sharing – talking it out with someone who is non-judgemental – can make you feel lighter. Each time you talk it out, it further reduces the hurt of the painful emotions associated with the traumatic event. This is the reason that people tend to share their ordeals with friends. It is the mind's natural coping mechanism. When you speak about matters of concern or pain, their imprint softens.

No imprint means no pain. No pain means you are healed. Healing of the mind is almost like returning to your original state of peace and bliss; of joy and happiness; of compassion and tolerance.

WITNESS MEDITATION – FOR MENTAL HEALTH

Thought is the energy through which you match or mismatch the frequency with the reality. Thought is an extraordinary force, and an average human brain is the playground of sixty thousand or so thoughts daily. There are some thoughts we hold on to and we pursue them. These can intrude upon our emotions and feelings, completely transforming them for better or worse.

Un-abandoned thoughts become desires, expectations or resolutions. They can give us direction or even misdirect us. The most important thing to remember, though, is that thoughts are devoid of any essence. In their own right, they have neither meaning nor value. It is what we do with thought that matters. On its own, the life of a thought is no more than a fraction of a second. It emerges, it manifests in our mind and it disappears. Between its emergence and disappearance is just a moment. If you do not react to the thought at that moment, it quietly goes away without disturbing your state of mind. Mostly, however, we grab hold of the thought, cling to it. A whole chain of interlinked thoughts follow and, before we know it, we are completely bogged down. A positive thought has a trail of positive thoughts and a negative thought has a trail of negative thoughts.

Witness meditation is the simple method of learning how not to react to your thoughts. If you have practised mindfulness, discussed in the next section, witness meditation is much easier. To do witness meditation, you don't need to be in the meditative posture, but it'll help if you are. So sit cross-legged if you can, or in a chair. Keep your head, neck and back in a straight line. Rest your hands in your lap if you are sitting cross-legged or on your knees if you are sitting in a chair. Take a few deep breaths, and think of yourself not as the doer or the maker of your life but simply as a witness.

Watch the thoughts as they come. Don't react to your thoughts: don't pursue them; don't reject them; don't accept them. Just watch them as if you are watching a movie. Let them be free; don't hold on to them. If it helps, think that these are the thoughts in the mind of someone you don't know. When thoughts of the past come, imagine that these thoughts don't belong to your own life but to some unknown person's life. Become a stranger to your own mind. Be completely indifferent to its flow of thoughts.

Steadily, you will see your thoughts slowing down, and you may also experience moments of complete cessation between them. If your own thoughts cannot provoke you, nothing external can provoke you either. Every external occurrence triggers an internal thought that may alter your state of mind. If you can just be the spectator and not the reactor or an adopter of the thought, the thought becomes powerless. You are taking the kinetic energy out of that thought, so it cannot bring a whole chain of thoughts with it. The thought will disappear right away.

Witness meditation helps you stay calm and stress-free – and resultantly physically fit. There will be no adrenaline rushes, no indigestion and no hypertension. You'll realize that you've always been an ocean of bliss, and no external force can move you.

MINDFULNESS – JOURNAL FOR EMOTIONAL HEALTH

A sage once asked his disciples, 'I have two bulls in my mind. One is eternally calm and happy. The other one is always restless and agitated. If the two go to fight, who will win?'

Some voted for the calm bull, arguing that calmness brings strength, while others vouched for the agitated one, saying that for fighting well, it is adrenaline that was needed.

'It depends,' the master said. 'Their victory depends on their strength. It is not necessary that one will always defeat the other. If you constantly feed the calm bull more than the angry one, it will grow stronger; its chances of winning every time go up.'

Mindfulness is one of the most powerful methods of improving your emotional health. It allows you to choose which of the two bulls you want to feed. The one you feed more often will win more frequently. Simply put, mindfulness is about being aware. When you feel negative, down, pensive, angry, sad, jealous and so forth, being mindful helps you emerge stronger than your negative emotions. It takes away the resistance and force from the negative emotions and you immediately feel better. If you are mindful, you can check the flow of thoughts; you can remind yourself that you do not wish to be negative or angry.

Just before you experience a surge of energy waiting to burst into words and actions, you have a moment to ponder over the choice you are about to exercise. You may gently remind yourself that you do not wish to let your blood boil – that you are not allowing negativity to get the better of you. Mindfulness transforms that fraction of a moment into peaceful contemplation; the juggernaut of negativity passes by.

As you cultivate the practice of mindfulness, you will find it increasingly easy to choose a preferred response in any situation. Often, a person's behaviour is governed by automatic responses. Someone yells at them and they either shout back or withdraw. This happens in a split second. They end up exercising a choice without realizing it. This is loss of mindfulness.

Writing a mindfulness journal is one of the best methods of starting to understand yourself. With this method, you identify your automatic responses and their triggers, so you may 'feed the calm bull' of mindfulness.

How to Do It

Each time you feel negative, agitated or indisposed, make a quick journal entry. It is best if you can do it right at that moment, but if you cannot, it is fine to do so after you have regained your composure. In your journal entry, answer the following four questions:

a. The episode: What was actually happening at the time you experienced negativity? Anything specific?
b. The cause: What triggered your negative emotion? Did someone say something or were you reminded of a past incident, for example?
c. The degree: To what extent did your negative emotion overpower you? For example, could you control yourself or did you end up doing something that you regretted later?

d. The future: Should a similar situation arise, would you respond in exactly the same manner, or would you respond differently?

If you wish to strengthen your practice even further, you may also journalize each time you are able to come out of your negative state. Writing a journal and reviewing it later helps you to analyse, understand and shape yourself better.

If you do not lose a sense of the present moment – if you remain committed to your inner peace – nothing can provoke you. Most negative emotions are symptomatic. They are not just emotions but emotional responses. With practice and mindfulness, you are able to choose your response better. Steadily, as you understand yourself better and learn to tame your stray emotions, you start to live in a state of inner quietude that is healing and empowering.

The resistance in your subtle body – in your emotions and in your inner self – starts to disappear and the resulting peaceful emotional state has a significant, noticeable and therapeutic effect on your physical body. This is what yogic texts call living in the sentiment of goodness (sattvic bhava).

There is little more to your physical, mental and emotional well-being than what you already know from reading this book. If you understand your constitution and choose your food accordingly, if you eat your food mindfully, if you understand your mind and choose your thoughts accordingly, if you regularly detoxify your physical and mental bodies, you will never need to visit a physician.

16

In a Nutshell

Let me give you the golden principle, the primordial mantra to stay in the finest of your physical, mental and emotional health. If you adopt what I am going to tell you, you will become a powerful agent – a catalyst in your own transformation. At the root of most ailments, diseases and disorder is clutter. Clutter could exist in your physical, mental or emotional world. Generally speaking, clutter in any one world is a strong indication that it also exists in the other two worlds.

Most of us carry a clutter of thoughts – often painful thoughts – of the past. We walk around in a mess of negative emotions, carrying a bag of unfulfilled desires. These thoughts and emotions continue to pile up, making us feel heavier and heavier, until one day we can take it no more and break down. This point of breakdown starts to manifest in the form of ailments in our three bodies – physical, mental and emotional – long before it appears in tests and medical imaging. How do we clean the clutter in the physical world? We organize the necessary stuff and discard the useless. This leads me to the golden mantra: simplify your life. This is truly the yogic sense, the wellness sense.

If you simplify your life, you will feel light and nourished. The easiest way to start simplifying your life is to de-clutter it. Start by cleaning up your physical world. Look around your study, your bedroom, your kitchen, your fridge and your garage. Get rid of as much stuff as you can and organize the rest. Make it a regular practice. This physical de-cluttering has a subtle effect on your mental state. The more you simplify your outer world, the greater the simplicity in the inner world. Use mindfulness and meditation as your tools to clean up your mental and emotional world as well.

Think about things of the past that cause you grief today: people you can't forgive, incidents you can't forget, feelings you can't let go of, thoughts you are holding on to and memories you are clinging to – all these and more that are adding to the emotional weight on you. It is time to discard them all. Write them down and shred the paper, letting go of them forever. Audit yourself minutely. These things are the real culprits; they are the agents of disease. They undermine the three doshas; it's these demons that weaken the seven dhatus. You can only benefit from destroying them. Simplify your life, diet, eating habits, thinking and living, and watch the miracles of wellness and joy unfold before your very eyes.

Here are some guiding principles to sum up everything that entails food and the eating sense:

- Eat wholesome foods as much as possible.
- All processed and canned fruits damage your health, therefore avoid them.

- Ideally, eighty per cent of your diet should consist of alkaline foods.
- Squeeze a fresh lemon or a half lemon in your glass of water whenever you can. It is a great antioxidant, highly alkaline and good for the skin too.
- Completely avoid fried foods.
- Think of artificial sweeteners as doses of poison.
- Chew your food well.
- Eat in moderation.
- Eat less than your stomach desires. Leave some room for air and water.
- Try to eat at the same time every day.
- Ideally, you should avoid eating after the sunset and in any case, your last meal of the day should be around four hours before you go to sleep.
- Avoid stale foods. According to Ayurveda, if three hours have elapsed since the food was cooked, it has turned stale. In modern terms, such food is oxidized and damaging for your health. Yogically, such food is tamasic and promotes ailments in the body.

Eating a good diet is mostly a common-sense matter. You need not be obsessed with numbers. Such obsession complicates life and we don't want that because, above all, it is simplification of life that yields the benefits of everything else.

Never go on a guilt trip. It is okay to break the rules of eating sense sometimes. If you are at a birthday party or a function and you are offered cake, rather than battling yourself to resist and dwelling on it, it's better to have a small piece. Thereafter, if you feel guilty, the same piece of cake will cause a lot more damage. Don't feel guilty; you have committed no crime. We are supposed to live and enjoy our lives, and food is one of the primary bases of our enjoyment. Treat yourself like an adult; treat yourself with care.

If you are mentally and emotionally positive and clear, and if you are free of stress, anomalies in diet can cause you practically no harm. Follow the principle of simplification in your decision making. No one needs to tell you what you should and shouldn't be eating or doing. When you consume food that is not good for you, it will have some cost to your health, energy and time. If you are willing to pay that price, by all means go ahead and have that food. Ultimately, you are your own best friend and your own worst enemy. You are the best judge when it comes to your own life.

Another matter that requires your attention is sleep. Sleeping is a divine gift. Our cells are repaired when we are sleeping. Nature allows us to forget our negative emotions, our painful thoughts, our past, our present and our future as it goes to work on our healing and rejuvenation. In the ideal world, everyone would take a short afternoon nap. If you are unable to have a siesta due to your work commitments, at least sleep really well at night. The easiest way to improve your sleep is to ensure that you sleep at the same time every day. If you change your sleeping time, you will often end up waking up in the middle of the night, only to look at the alarm clock. When you sleep at the same time every day, your body falls into a perfect rhythm. It becomes more efficient at executing the repair and healing processes while you sleep. Plus, you won't need an alarm clock to wake up in the morning – your body already has an 'atomic clock'.

To optimize the quality of your sleep, you need to consider your sleeping position, and your optimal sleeping position depends on your dosha. It is best to sleep to your left if you are a kapha. When you sleep on the left side, the right nostril opens up for breathing. The right breath is called the solar breath. It generates heat in the body. If you are a pitta, you are best to sleep on your right side, because sleeping on the right activates your lunar breath from the left nostril, which maintains a sort of coolness in the body. A vata may sleep on either side. These are not set-in-stone rules: in all likelihood, you will change your position after falling asleep, anyway. If sometimes you can't avoid having a late dinner and have to go to bed before it's digested, it's better to sleep to your left side, so it ignites the digestive fire.

This is the day and age of distractions – twenty-four-hour television channels, Internet, social media and cellphones – and this ultra-connectivity and activity rob you of quality time. Whatever you do, moderation is worth practising. If we were to sum up Ayurveda in one word, it would probably be moderation. Balance is the key. Once in a while you may indulge, but if you let things come in the way of balanced living, they start to overtake your life. And one day, before you know it, those aspects are ruling your life; they are consuming you, rather than the other way round.

Finally, never fail to express your gratitude for all you have been blessed with. This is the easiest way of summoning nature – of becoming one with it. Every object on our planet and in our universe has an impact on our lives, however tiny it may be. Think about this: the moon, a celestial object devoid of any life, is more than 234,000 miles away, and yet it can cause massive tides in the oceans on earth. The strong gravitational pull of the earth cannot stop those tides. Can we reasonably assume that the full moon that is causing the oceans to swell is having no impact on us? I don't think so. The effect might be subtle, but it does not mean it's insignificant.

As we become more evolved, emotionally and spiritually, we become more sensitive; we notice and feel more. Astrological treatises assign various foods to various days. And they state that the fertility and sexual drive of a woman is directly linked to the moon, for example. My point is that we are more than the sum total of the three doshas and seven dhatus. We contain within ourselves an entire universe. The more natural our lives, the healthier we become. When our frequency matches that of nature's, diseases can no longer exist in our bodies. If living physically close to nature is not possible, eating natural foods is the next best thing you can do. If you don't forget that everything springs from energy, and there's no true structural reality, you can remain eternally healthy. Such an understanding will lead you to the right thought and right action, and right consequences will follow.

Your health is in your hands. It starts and ends with you.

Appendices

Appendix 1
Acidic and Alkaline Foods

It's not the pH level of the food itself but its effect on digestion that is most significant. In other words, it's not just the taste (rasa) of the food that matters when it comes to acidity/alkalinity but the post-digestive state (vipaka) and overall effect (prabhava). The tables below factor all three.

Alkaline Foods

Highly Alkaline and Sattvic	Moderately Alkaline and Rajasic	Slightly Alkaline and Tamasic
Vegetables	**Vegetables**	**Vegetables**
Asparagus	Alfalfa	Fermented veggies
Bottle gourd	Artichokes	Garlic
Broccoli	Barley grass	Mushrooms
Brussels sprouts	Beetroot	Mustard greens
Cauliflower	Cabbage	Onions
Celery	Carrot	Parsnips
Cucumber	Ginger	Radish

Highly Alkaline and Sattvic	Moderately Alkaline and Rajasic	Slightly Alkaline and Tamasic
Vegetables	**Vegetables**	**Vegetables**
Dandelions	Green beans and	Sea vegetables
Eggplant	soya bean	Spirulina
Kale	Kale	Turnip
Lemons	Mustard greens	Watercress
Lettuce	Okra	
Potato	Peas	
Pumpkin	Peppers	
Spinach	Sprouts	
Squashes	Wheat grass	
Sweet potato	Green olives	
Watercress		
Fruits	**Fruits**	**Fruits**
Avocado	Apples	Grapefruit
Fresh Coconut	Banana	Grapes
Lime	Blackberries	Raspberries
Mango	Cherries	Rhubarb
Papaya	Peaches	Strawberries
	Pears	Watermelon
	Tomato	
Others	**Others**	**Others**
Ghee from cow milk	All sprouts	Herbal teas
Water from natural spring or RO system	Ghee from buffalo milk	
	Butter	
	Olive oil	
	Most spices	

Note: Ideally, the majority of your diet should consist of alkaline foods.

Acidic Foods

Slightly Acidic and Sattvic	*Moderately Acidic and Rajasic*	*Highly Acidic and Tamasic*
Vegetables	**Vegetables**	**Vegetables**
Black olives	Black beans	Soybeans
Chickpeas	Corn	
Spinach		
Fruits		
Apricots		
Dates		
Figs		
Guava		
Others	**Others**	**Others**
Brown rice	Black tea	Artificial sweeteners
Brown sugar	Bottled juices	Beef
Cow milk	Buffalo's milk	Beer
Fresh juices	Cheese	Carbonated soft
Normal tap water	Coffee	drinks
Vegetable oil	Flavoured milk	Chicken
White rice	Ice creams	Cocoa
Wholewheat bread	Most dry fruits	Eggs
Wholewheat pasta	Peanuts	Jam
	Red wine	Liquor
	Sea salt	Mayonnaise
	Table salt	Most fried foods
	White bread	Most sauces
	White pasta	Pork
	White sugar	Seafood
	White Wine	Turkey
		Vinegar
		Vodka
		Whisky
		Yeast

Notes:

All processed foods and fast foods are highly acidic.

All breads and pastas made from white flour are acidic and rajasic.

All forms of poultry, meat and alcohol are highly acidic and tamasic.

All bottled or canned sauces and carbonated drinks are highly acidic.

Most wholesome foods are either sattvic or alkali-forming.

Organic foods are far better than non-organic foods.

Chlorinated water is acidic.

A healthy diet has at least eighty per cent alkaline foods.

From the Ayurvedic perspective, the more sattvic food you eat, the healthier your diet.

Eat as much as you can from the left side of this chart. The foods on the left of the chart are more nourishing than those in the middle and on the right.

Appendix 2
The Five Sheaths

The five elements in our bodies directly affect the state of the five sheaths and vice versa. The five sheaths represent various anatomical, physiological, psychical, intellectual and transcendental elements and processes that influence every aspect of our existence. From the union of an egg with a sperm till one's last breath, there is a reciprocal relationship between these sheaths and our thoughts, emotions and actions. How we conduct our lives affects the sheaths and these sheaths, in turn, dictate our emotional and physical health. They are the five aspects of your whole being. See the table below:

The Five Sheaths and Elements

Element	Sheath	Sanskrit Term
Earth	Anatomical	Annamaya kosha
Water	Physiological	Pranamaya kosha
Fire	Psychical	Manomaya kosha
Air	Intellectual	Vijnanamaya kosha
Ether	Transcendental	Anandamaya kosha

The first sheath is dominated by the earth element and is called the anatomical sheath. The Sanskrit term is annamaya kosha. Anna means food; kosha means sheath. Your physical body is the sum total of materials formed by consuming food. From the formation of an embryo to surviving in the outside world, your body is a direct result of what you eat.

Weakness in the anatomical sheath creates diseases linked to the earth element. These could be as simple as acne and muscle aches, to more complicated benign lumps in the body requiring surgical removal. The food you eat has a direct and noticeable effect on your body. That being said, without the biological processes, there is no functioning; we are as good as dead. And this leads to the second sheath.

Even more important than the anatomical sheath, the second sheath has a direct impact on your physical health. It is called the physiological sheath (pranamaya kosha). Prana means the vital life force. It also means energy. There are five primary energies in your body. These are known as the five pranas (see Appendix 4). They are constantly flowing. If they cease to flow, there will be no breathing, digestion, excretions, secretions or speech.

The body ceases to function in the absence of these vital energies. A dead body, even though anatomically complete, can only rot. The vital energies keep the body alive. The five primary energies and the five secondary ones comprising the physiological sheath are covered in more detail in the following pages (Appendix 4). Deficiencies in the physiological sheath causes diseases related to the water element. They could range from excess urination to blood cancer.

The third sheath is the psychical sheath (manomaya kosha). A body may have an energy flow, it may be living, but without its psychic faculties it will be a vegetable. The literal meaning of manomaya is 'made up of mind'. By psychic faculties, I don't mean anything mystical or abstract but simply our mental processes. The psychical sheath can't exist on its own, because a brain can only function if it is receiving oxygen. Therefore, the health and quality of the physiological sheath have a direct bearing on your mental health. The psychical sheath governs the fire element. Any holes in this sheath can result in anything from indigestion to stupor to malignant tumours in the physical body.

Every living creature, certainly any animate one, has three sheaths. From ants to an elephant, all animals have these three sheaths. But we have a special utility of the elements of air and ether that gives us two additional sheaths.

We are much more evolved than animals because of these two additional sheaths. The fourth is the intellectual sheath (vijnanamaya kosha). When our consciousness connects with the three sheaths, it gives birth to discriminating faculties of the mind. Our minds are able to discriminate between right and wrong. We can create information. We can hypothesize. We can assess and reach intellectual conclusions. We can perceive future threats; we can meditate and contemplate. This – the functioning of the intellectual sheath – is what makes us human.

With the help of this sheath, we can dream of a future and put our intelligence to use. It gives us the capacity for rational thought and inference. All living beings have intelligence, but only humans have intellect. The fourth sheath is linked to the air element. All mental disorders, from clinical depression to schizophrenia, are connected to this sheath and its corresponding element.

The first four sheaths – while they create us and affect

us – are merely a covering on the one that really matters. These four sheaths make us forget our true selves – our intrinsic natures. Caught and torn between their biological, mental and emotional needs, most people spend their whole lives in a state of disequilibrium. Most of our fellow humans grow up, get a degree, get a job, get married, have kids, look after them, keep working, retire, get old and die. The beautiful life we are meant to celebrate is often wasted in meaningless pursuits, unfulfilled expectations, grudges, complaints, negativity and the rest. These pursuits are not wrong; our emotions are natural. But the truth is that they cover the real you. The first four sheaths don't define who you really are.

There is more to you. The fifth sheath is called the transcendental sheath (anandamaya kosha). Its literal meaning is a sheath of bliss. Your true nature transcends the shackles of the body, the flow of energies, the limitations of the mind and the conditioning of intellect: you are beyond these. You are an ocean of bliss. Sometimes, when you get glimpses of your true nature, you feel euphoric and infinite. This fifth transcendental sheath is beyond debilitation, diseases and disorders. It is a state of pure bliss.

The five great elements and the five sheaths segregate our existence into three parts. This is not gross division but a yogic framework to better utilize human potential. These three parts are called the three bodies. We have a gross body, a subtle body and a causal body. This is detailed in Appendix 3.

Appendix 3
The Three Bodies

On the surface, it may appear that you have a physical body, and its health is directly dependent on how you keep it and what you feed it. While this is not untrue, it is not the complete truth; it is not even half the truth. Just like a tiny cellphone allows us to make and receive calls, the structure of the cellphone alone does not give us the full picture. There is an electrical charge in it and a SIM card. It is communicating with the cellphone tower, which in turn communicates through a satellite. Think of your physical body as the cellphone. The software in it is your subtle body, and the electrical charge is the causal body. All three are needed for any communication to occur, and it's practically of no use if we can't make or take calls. Even with the three present, there needs to be a communication tower, a satellite – some infrastructure. Similarly, the three bodies are constantly impacted by the environment around us. Let me elucidate the three bodies.

Physical Body

Yogic texts call it sthula sharira. Sthula means gross, carnal or physical and sharira means body. It is also called karya sharira. Karya means duty or action. We perform all actions through this body. Your anatomical body is your physical body, and it is made up of the five elements and the seven tissues (covered later in this appendix). It includes your cognitive, conative and vital organs. It is through the physical body alone that you can perform any physical action. It is your field of karma. This is the first sheath. You eat and process food through your physical body. This body is perishable, though. Its only truth is death – it is ever deteriorating. Everyone is getting older.

Modern medical science treats the physical body as the cause and the consequence. Ayurveda and yogic texts approach it very differently. Any disease appearing in your physical body is generally not the cause but merely a symptom of an underlying problem. The problem has got out of hand and has expressed itself in your physical body, generally in the form of a disorder. Such disorders could range from simple allergies to terminal diseases; they could be anything from indigestion to chronic diabetes. The physical body in itself is not the originator – it is merely the messenger. Doubtless, there are some things you simply can't change about your body but the rest of it, which is most of it – health and well-being included – remains entirely in your hands.

SUBTLE BODY

Your subtle body comprises three of the five sheaths. They are physiological, psychical and intellectual sheaths. It is called sukshma sharira or the linga sharira. Sukshma means subtle. In various sutras and Vedic philosophical treatises, there is an important and revealing definition of the word linga. It means the invisible mark that proves the existence of something; a mark that is inherent evidence. For thousands of years, Shivalingam has been worshipped in India. Shivalingam is an elongated cylindrical structure, rounded at the top, on an elliptical base. It is carved out of one stone. The top represents the masculine principle; it corresponds to the seed of creation. It is also called Purusha, the Supreme Man.

The word Purusha also means the One who has entered into the city of nine gates. This body is called a pura (city) of nine gates. The nine gates are the nine orifices of the human body (ten in the case of a female). The base of the Shivalingam represents the feminine principle; it means sustenance. It is also called Prakriti. Prakriti means Mother Nature, but it also means your constitution. Your constitution is the basis of Ayurveda. Shiva is the destroyer in the Vedic pantheon. This exemplifies the fundamental truth that seeds of destruction are present in the very creation – and sustenance – of every physical element. Creation, sustenance and destruction are simply three indivisible facets of existence.

And creation, sustenance and destruction are the three constant aspects of your bodily existence. To maintain the best health, your body undergoes degeneration and regeneration at the cellular level. For example, red blood cells meet their destruction every one hundred and twenty days and the bone marrow produces new blood cells. The development of spermatozoa takes seventy-one days, and they are destroyed within five days of ejaculation. Ova, the female reproductive cells, are only available for thirty-six hours. Every secretion in our bodies – everything about us, even the tiniest facet of our existence – has its own life cycle. Nature knows this.

Your subtle body is the one that sustains the flow of various energies: your consciousness and your intellect. It governs the physiology of the physical body. In its absence, the physical body is dead, and the only possibilities for a dead body are decomposition and disintegration. The subtle body is invisible, but it has a direct influence on your physical and mental well-being. If you take care of the subtle body, your physical health improves automatically and even dramatically. When the subtle body is healthy, any food you consume is properly processed by the body; the food nourishes you.

CAUSAL BODY

The causal body is called karana sharira in Sanskrit. It is the cause on which the other two bodies rest. The causal body relates to your true and original nature of peace and bliss. Vedic texts state that your atman (soul) is above the three bodies, and that the causal body refers to your original state of bliss. To keep things simple, however, think of the causal body as your soul. When a person dies, he is unable to respond to any stimulation. Why? Because the causal body (the soul) has gone, and therefore the subtle body cannot operate either. Hence the physical body is already dead.

When you nourish and nurture your physical and subtle bodies, you feel more and more connected with your soul. The more you work on self-purification, the more bliss you enjoy in life.

Appendix 4
The Ten Energies

The ten energies control all voluntary and involuntary physical actions, reactions and habits. The energies, in turn, can be controlled by asana siddhi – mastery of the yogic posture, regulation of the breath and concentrative meditation. The Sanskrit term is vayu. It means fluid, subtle energy. It is a term frequently used to mean wind as well. The ten vital energies are divided into five primary and five secondary energies. Their functions are as follows.

PRIMARY ENERGIES

1. Prana vayu or vital life energy: This energy is the basis of your life. It is the vital life force in your breath, the subtle element in oxygen. It is almost like fuel for your body. It has a direct impact on your state of mind, your emotions, moods and disposition.

2. Apana vayu or descending energy: Urine, seminal fluids and defecation are controlled by the descending energy. It predominantly lives below your stomach. Mastery over this vayu can give you control over urination, bowel movements and ejaculation.

3. Udana vayu or ascending energy: This energy lives in your throat and is responsible for producing the voice. Thyroid glands can be controlled by the manipulation of ascending energy. Thyroid glands directly affect the production of hormones.

4. Samana vayu or thermal energy: This energy resides in your stomach. It is responsible for the movement of food and digestion. Control of this energy can help you change your body heat at will. Channelled thermal energy will give you an exceptionally well-functioning colon and metabolism.

5. Vyana vayu or diffusive energy: This energy circulates through your whole body. It causes the blood to transport oxygen to all parts of the body. Manipulation of this energy can help you stay in one posture for as long as you want.

SECONDARY ENERGIES

1. Naga: It controls belching, burping and all upwards wind movement from your stomach.

2. Kurma: It controls sneezing and all abnormal wind movement in the sinuses.

3. Krikara: It controls the blinking of the eyes.

4. Devadatta: Yawning can be completely controlled by manipulation of this vayu.

5. Dhananjaya: Twitching in any part of the body is affected by this energy.

There are many yogic practices aimed at stilling the ten energies. Stillness of the ten energies infuses extraordinary calmness and willpower in the practitioner.

Further Reading

If you are interested in knowing more about Ayurveda and yoga, I recommend you read the following classical texts. Many learned ones have translated them and I don't have any personal favourites per se, so pick any translation you like. I read most of these texts nearly two decades ago but I am naming these here because they are the basis of my theoretical exposition in this book:

- *Sharangdhara Samhita*
- *Sushurta Samhita*
- *Charaka Samhita*
- *Bhavprakash Nighantu*
- *Harita Samhita*
- *Kashyapa Samhita*
- *Ashtanga Samgraha*
- *Ashtanga Hridayam*
- *Shiva Samhita*
- *Gheranda Samhita*
- *Hatha Yoga Pradipika*

- *Rasa Tattva Chintamani* (no English translation available, I believe)
- *Rasaratna Samuchchaya* (no English translation available, I believe)

Other than the classical texts cited above, I came across some wonderful writings in the past few years. Parts of this book have been influenced by the thoughts of these scholars. You too will gain much from reading the following:

- *Light on the Yoga Sutras of Patanjali* by B.K.S. Iyengar
- *Light on Life: The Yoga Journey to Wholeness, Inner Peace, and Ultimate Freedom* by B.K.S. Iyengar
- *Prakriti: Your Ayurvedic Constitution* by Robert E. Svoboda
- A translation of *Charaka Samhita* by Gabriel van Loon
- *The Acid Alkaline Food Guide* by Dr Susan Brown and Larry Triveri Jr
- *The Enzyme Factor* by Hiromi Shinya

With some research, you should be able to get your hands on almost all of these.

Also by Om Swami

If Truth Be Told – A Monk's Memoir

A HarperCollins imprint

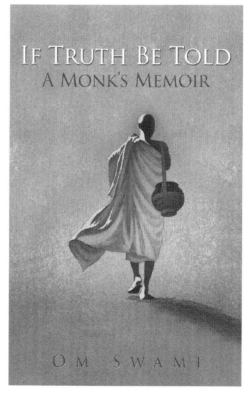

Go to omswami.com for more.

Printed in Great Britain
by Amazon

63312441R00142